ENJOY FOODS WITH... ...OUR
LOSE WEIGHT FO...

THE SONOMA DIET™

Trimmer waist, better health in just 10 days!

WWW.SONOMADIET.COM

MICHAEL JOSEPH
an imprint of
PENGUIN BOOKS

DR CONNIE GUTTERSEN, R.D., PH.D.

MICHAEL JOSEPH

Published by the Penguin Group
Penguin Books Ltd, 80 Strand, London WC2R 0RL, England
Penguin Group (USA) Inc., 375 Hudson Street, New York, New York 10014, USA
Penguin Group (Canada), 90 Eglinton Avenue East, Suite 700, Toronto, Ontario, Canada M4P 2Y3
(a division of Pearson Penguin Canada Inc.)
Penguin Ireland, 25 St Stephen's Green, Dublin 2, Ireland (a division of Penguin Books Ltd)
Penguin Group (Australia), 250 Camberwell Road,Camberwell, Victoria 3124, Australia
(a division of Pearson Australia Group Pty)
Penguin Books India Pvt Ltd, 11 Community Centre, Panchsheel Park, New Delhi – 110 017, India
Penguin Group (NZ), cnr Airborne and Rosedale Roads, Albany, Auckland 1310, New Zealand
(a division of Pearson New Zealand Ltd)
Penguin Books (South Africa) (Pty) Ltd, 24 Sturdee Avenue, Rosebank, Johannesburg 2196, South Africa

Penguin Books Ltd, Registered Offices: 80 Strand, London WC2R 0RL, England

www.penguin.com

First published in the USA by Meredith Books 2005
First published in Great Britain by Michael Joseph 2006
1

Printed in England by Clays Ltd, St Ives plc

ISBN-13: 978–0–718–14926–0
ISBN-10: 0–718–14926–2

SEE YOUR DOCTOR FIRST

This diet book is designed to provide helpful information on the subjects addressed.
This book is sold with the understanding that the author and publisher are not
rendering medical, health, or other personal services. Please consult your personal
physician before commencing the Sonoma Diet and also before changing your diet
or exercise routine. You should rely on your physician's advice regarding whether
the Sonoma Diet is appropriate for you and you should rely on your physician to
establish your weight goal. The author and publisher disclaim all liability associated
with the recommendations and guidelines set forth in this book.

The Sonoma Diet is a trademark of Meredith Corporation.

Acknowledgements

I would like to thank the Sonoma Diet team for their knowledge, time, and effort: Bob Mate, Jim Blume, Doug Guendel, Patrick Taylor, Jennifer Darling, Stephanie Karpinske, Amy Nichols, Gina Rickert, Steve Rogers, Jeff Myers, Greg Kayko, Margie Schenkelberg, Matt Strelecki, Ken Carlson, Som Inthalangsy, Andy Lyons, Faith Echtermeyer, and Laura Harms. Thank you to Kelly Garret for his professional and accurate approach to writing. A special thanks to Heidi Krupp for her invaluable experience. Jeremy Woolf, Jennifer Ull, and the rest of the Krupp Gang—everything you do is in great taste!

I would like to acknowledge Chef Toni Hendrickson Sakaguchi for her culinary inspiration in this project and my friends at the Culinary Institute of America at Greystone who have taught me to include flavour and enjoyment as part of nutrition. Also, sincere thanks to Dr Mark Dedomenico, in Bellevue, Washington, for his encouragement to continue my endeavours in the treatment of obesity and its related diseases.

I am indebted to my late father, Bruno Peraglie, M.D., and brother, Cesare Peraglie, M.D., a fourth-generation physician. Thank you for exposing me to the importance of nutrition, well-being, and the responsibility that each of us has in maintaining our own health. I am grateful to my husband, Shawn, and our children, Gabriella and William, for their motivation and support in this project.

Publisher's Note

For the benefit of readers in the UK, the original US measurements in this book have been converted. As a result, the figures in the Nutrition Facts at the end of each recipe should be regarded as approximate rather than exact.

From the Author

I strongly believe that flavourful food is the missing element to the long-term success of any diet. The Sonoma Diet is based on one of the most flavourful cuisines in the world—the foods of the Mediterranean, which are not only delicious, but also have health benefits. Today, as I work at the Culinary Institute of America in California's wine country, I'm immersed in the world of flavour and its effect on how and what we eat. The cuisine of the sun-drenched Sonoma and Napa Valleys is its own interpretation of the Mediterranean diet. It celebrates fresh ingredients, wholesome food, and an eating style where meals are leisurely enjoyed.

My interest in food and health began very early. I come from generations of medical doctors who believed good nutrition was key to good health. After earning my Ph.D. in nutrition, I worked as a nutrition professor at Texas Christian University. Then I spent 10 years counselling people struggling with obesity and weight management. Through my patients I started to see the many frustrations with weight-loss programmes. It really hit home when my own father became overweight and got stuck in the dieting cycle. I gained insight and compassion for dieters as I saw him suffer through the deprivation, the tasteless food, and the experience of drinking a chalky diet shake while everyone else at the table ate "real" food. It was clear to me then that there was a key element missing in today's "diets."

The philosophy behind the Sonoma Diet, which has been in the making for many years, is based on a variety of scientific studies. Through my own nutrition expertise, I've taken these findings and translated them into a diet that gives you long-term weight loss and a healthier life. I've also worked with top chefs to develop fresh, flavourful recipes that make this diet unique. So when you see the words "we" throughout this book, I'm referring to the researchers, culinary experts, and other people who have educated and inspired me, both indirectly and directly, to create the Sonoma Diet.

The Sonoma Diet can be your way of losing weight and gaining a healthy lifestyle. Here's to good food, successful weight loss, and healthier living.

The Sonoma Diet

TABLE OF CONTENTS

WELCOME TO YOUR NEW LIFESTYLE

The Sonoma Diet is like no other.

You will lose every ounce of excess weight that you need to. But at the same time, you will enjoy eating more than you ever have in your life. It is a way of eating where meals are a celebration, not deprivation.

That's because on the Sonoma Diet, you don't lose weight by avoiding food. Instead, you lose weight by enjoying satisfying amounts of the best foods on the planet. Perhaps for the first time in your life, you will truly cherish your meals. The Sonoma Diet celebrates the food and flavour renaissance that is happening across America today.

There's no "diet food" on the Sonoma Diet. No specialty foods. Nothing out of the ordinary. Just wholesome, fresh, and delicious everyday foods that are easy to find and even easier to prepare.

The results are phenomenal. You'll shed pounds quickly at first, then steadily until your weight is right where you always wanted it to be (and maybe never dared to hope it could be!). And it's weight loss that lasts a lifetime.

Every step of your journey from overweight to perfect weight will be comfortable, pleasant, and simple. Enjoy the same food with everyone else at the table. You won't have to track calories, keep score of any "points," or constantly weigh and measure your food. Forget about eating different foods from everybody else around you. You'll barely remember you're on a diet.

We've done all the science for you, down to the last nutritional detail. So you don't have to count, plan, analyse, or worry. All you have to do is select from a huge variety of food choices, then follow our guidelines. Use the recipes we give you if you like. But the main thing is, enjoy your meals.

The Sonoma Diet also offers what other diets tend to ignore—a healthier and more energetic you. Sure, if you're overweight, weight loss itself will help your health. But the Sonoma Diet offers much more than that. With this plan, improved health isn't just a side effect of weight loss. It is the very route to weight loss. You will feel your new health and energy well before you lose that last pound.

Too good to be true? On the contrary, the Sonoma Diet is based on the very latest discoveries about nutrition, health, and weight loss. Behind every meal plan and food recommendation is cutting-edge research that goes beyond the now-dated notions of low-carb or low-fat. You will fill up on "power foods" that deliver maximum disease-fighting nutrients with a minimum of calories. You'll be eating meals in carefully planned combinations that not only bring out hidden flavours but also maximize your body's absorption of essential nutrients.

These power combos are at the heart of the Sonoma Diet. They're a big reason you'll be discovering a new vibrant health as well as a slimmer shape. Think about it. Shouldn't a diet give you both of those things? Nothing else makes sense.

In fact, you'll be emulating the Mediterranean way of eating, famous for limiting heart disease and prolonging life among the southern Europeans— as well as keeping them trim. A Mediterranean meal is a feast for the senses and a boon for health and longevity. That's exactly how you're going to eat on the Sonoma Diet.

Most important for your success, you'll feel pleased and satisfied all day long. The Sonoma Diet does not invite frustration by artificially limiting any category of food. That makes it the perfect "next-step" diet for everyone who's tried and failed to stick to a "low-carb" or "low-fat" diet. The Sonoma Diet is not "low" anything. It is a balanced meal plan that provides your body everything it needs.

The Sonoma Diet is not a deprivation diet. Meat, fish, beans, eggs—they're all there for you. Snacks? Of course. Wine? Sure, if you like. In moderation, it's good for you.

Instead of banning whole categories of foods, the Sonoma Diet helps you eat reasonable amounts of the leanest, healthiest foods in each category. You'll learn to satisfy your hunger without overeating. You'll learn to eat slowly and savour every bite. And you'll learn how to finish a meal feeling content, never deprived.

The Sonoma Diet is not a low-carb diet. On the contrary, it stresses a huge variety of plant-based, carbohydrate-rich energy food. Do you like rice or other grains with your main course? Enjoy them, as long as they're the best-tasting, whole grain, fibre-rich version. Bread? You bet, and from Day 1 of your diet. Cereals? Every day if you like. Fruits and vegetables? In abundance.

The Sonoma Diet is not a low-fat diet, either. Heart-healthy and flavour-enhancing olive oil can be an everyday feature of your meals, bringing out nutrients and flavours in many of the foods you eat.

You'll be encouraged to take advantage of other healthy dietary fats as well. A variety of nuts and avocados, for example, and the heart-protective natural oils in fish will help you lose weight and keep you satisfied as you do it.

The Sonoma Diet's secret to weight loss is rediscovering the "right way to eat." It's about the sensual joy of savouring a variety of fresh, wholesome, and delicious foods. In other words, you'll be adopting a new eating lifestyle. You'll find it far more pleasurable and satisfying than the one you'll be leaving behind. The Sonoma Diet lifestyle will be a part of you long after you've reached your target weight. It will keep you slim, healthy, and enjoying every meal for the rest of your life.

It's a diet you can live with.

THE SONOMA REGION

How did the diet get its name? That's an excellent question, because the name "Sonoma" is synonymous with the spirit of the diet you'll be following. To understand it, we need to do a little elementary geography work.

Pull out a world map and find the Mediterranean Sea. Trace your finger along the sea's perimeter and notice what you cross—among other places, you'll pass through coastal Spain, southern France, Italy, Greece.

What are these lands known for? Ideal climates, fresh fruits and vegetables, fine wines, lean meats, abundant fish, and heart-friendly olive oil. In fact, the eating habits and the active lifestyle in this part of the world are so beneficial to human health that science has a name for it—the Mediterranean diet.

Now stick your finger in the middle of Italy and follow the line straight westward across the Atlantic and the United States until you come to the California coast. You're in Sonoma County, north of San Francisco Bay.

Here the waves break on rocky coasts that give way to majestic redwood forests covering coastal mountains. Further inland, rolling hills are dotted with olive trees and apple groves.

On countless slopes lie some of the most lauded vineyards in the world, the grapes gleaming green and purple in the California sun. Along Sonoma's rustic trails and rural back roads, hikers and cyclists exercise as they take in the beauty of the surroundings.

This breathtakingly scenic region shares more in common with the Mediterranean than latitude and climate. Its fruits and vegetables are just as fresh and delicious, its wine as fine, its meat as lean, its fish and other seafood as abundant, its homegrown olive oil just as heart-friendly. The lifestyle? Even healthier.

Out of the farms and restaurants and kitchens of this idyllic home of healthy, sensuous eating comes the Sonoma Diet.

It is a Western Hemisphere version of the Mediterranean diet. Therefore, it lowers your risk of heart disease and certain cancers and offers you a longer, more active, more rewarding life.

The people of southern Europe and Sonoma contributed the element of pleasure to the diet. We've added another benefit: safe, permanent weight loss.

WEIGHT LOSS PLUS DELICIOUS FOODS

The emphasis of the Sonoma Diet, to repeat, is not to avoid good food but to eat the best foods on the planet. Here are some of them:

Lots of the best fresh fruits and vegetables instead of processed foods and sugary sweets. Generous allotments of whole grain bread and cereals instead of refined white flour products. Skinless white meat poultry, lean red meats, lamb, pork, veal, eggs, non-fat dairy, soya beans, and plenty of fish for your protein. Olive oil and nuts as your main dietary fat sources. Unlimited herbs and spices. A little wine. It doesn't matter if you live in Los Angeles, Dallas, New York, Seattle, or Denver. The Sonoma Diet can be your "way of eating."

Sound appealing? Then you're already in the spirit of the Sonoma Diet.

The chapters that follow will take you through the diet step-by-step. The first thing you'll notice is how simple everything is. There's no rule that says good eating has to be complicated.

After a summary of the major points of the diet, you'll be introduced to the huge variety of foods you'll be eating. The emphasis will be on the power foods that deliver the most health-imparting nutrients with the fewest calories.

Then you'll be guided through the diet itself, with specific instructions on choosing foods, preparing them, and eating them in the right proportions and amounts. You'll find recipes, specific meals to prepare, and specific tips for making things easy and for getting the most from your diet.

There are also chapters dedicated to helping you through the inevitable rough spots—the cravings, the hurdles, the frustrations that pop up from time to time on any diet. We'll tell you exactly how to deal with any problem, so you can leave it behind and move on to your weight loss goal.

Within days of starting the Sonoma Diet, you'll already notice a change for the better in the way you feel and the way your clothes fit. You will begin losing weight immediately.

You'll also notice a difference in the way you think about food. As you leave the old bad ways behind and adopt the new good ways, you'll discover an amazing thing. The new way tastes better! You're feeling better, you're losing weight—and you're enjoying your meals more than you ever thought possible.

That's what the Sonoma Diet is all about. Let's get started.

WHAT IS THE SONOMA DIET?

The Sonoma Diet is a unique weight loss plan that, for the first time, brings together the art and science of food. The appreciation and enjoyment of flavourful meals makes for a healthy eating style that becomes second nature. Simple guidelines for the amount and combinations of food make the plate your guide. This was all designed for you to shed pounds safely and easily until you reach your best body weight.

The foods and recipes that will get you there have been carefully selected to make you healthier and happier as you lose the weight. The latest knowledge from the fast-evolving world of nutritional research is reflected in the food selection and meal preparations.

But this diet wasn't born in a lab.

Its true creators are the vitality-radiating residents of two special places in the real world, places where the intense enjoyment of an abundance of delicious food is a way of life. The Sonoma Diet gets its name from one of these places. It is inspired by the great-tasting, sun-drenched foods that make California's beautiful Sonoma County a paradise of healthy eating and active lifestyles.

Sonoma cuisine, in turn, is a state of mind and reflection of the "way of eating" and daily foods enjoyed by the people who live on or near the Mediterranean Sea. The southern Europeans who live this "Mediterranean diet" enjoy a bounty of wholesome and delicious fresh foods, including vegetables, whole grains, nuts, olive oil, lean meats, and wine. Sonoma cuisine, with its diverse flavours and local fare, is its own unique interpretation of the Mediterranean diet.

These two communities—New World and Old World—have something in common besides superb nutritional instincts. They share a festive approach to eating, a heartfelt love of great food that turns every meal into a celebration of life.

You'll feel that same joy of eating because it's at the core of the Sonoma Diet. In fact, savouring the flavours and wide selection of recipes is essential to your success. When we say "enjoy your meal," we really mean it.

FRESH FROM THE MEDITERRANEAN

Decades ago, researchers started pondering a seeming paradox. Why is it that Mediterranean populations live healthier, longer lives with lower rates of heart disease, cancer, obesity, and diabetes compared to many parts of the world? When Americans or northern Europeans eat what they consider pleasurable feasts, they're told they're raising their heart attack risk. When southern Europeans eat their versions of the same thing, they get healthier. What's going on?

The answer lies in the flavourful, nutrient-rich foods and "way of living" of the Mediterranean diet. It exemplifies the cornerstones of healthy eating. Minimal processing and seasonal choices maximize the content of nutrients in these foods. Health is not based on avoiding certain "danger" or "unhealthy" foods; it is about enjoying more of those foods that are nutrient rich.

The Sonoma Diet is based exactly on that healthy inspiration for selecting foods. It emphasizes eating a generous variety of foods that boost your vitality, protect your heart, and improve your overall health. Most of those foods are the same ones that dominate the Mediterranean diet.

What does the Mediterranean diet consist of? It is a variety of different cuisines, from southern Italy, Spain, Morocco, Tunisia, Greece, and southern France. These cuisines contribute their own flavour palates but maintain a common thread—olives, grapes, and wheat. The dishes are largely plant-based, which means seasonal vegetables, whole grains, fruits, beans, nuts, and olive oil play leading roles. Olive oil goes beyond health benefits—it provides flavour for the enjoyment of large quantities of vegetables and legumes in salads and other dishes. (This offers an important lesson. Perhaps you don't eat enough vegetables and legumes because you haven't learned how to prepare them in flavourful ways.) Fish and poultry are more prominent than red meat or dairy. Wine, red or white, also plays an important role in the meal. Foods are simple, unpretentious, and flavoured with herbs and spices.

In fact, you'll be eating much as you would in the Mediterranean in the sense that you'll be taking advantage of health-boosting foods as much as possible. We call these "Power Foods." They deliver maximum nutrition with minimum calories. Eating these miracles of nature is as important for weight loss as not eating "fattening" foods.

The Sonoma Factor

The Sonoma Diet may be based nutritionally on the healthy eating habits of the Mediterranean countries, but it's inspired by Sonoma County's culinary creativity and love of fresh, wholesome, great-tasting foods.

The biggest difference between the Sonoma and Mediterranean diets, though, is the goal. The Sonoma Diet is designed for you to lose weight. The Mediterranean diet is not. The word "diet" after the word "Mediterranean" simply refers to what is eaten every day. The word "diet" after "Sonoma" refers to a weight-loss programme.

The Sonoma Diet, then, is an adjustment of the Mediterranean diet to include weight-loss strategies based on the most up-to-date knowledge about what works and what doesn't. It

See Your Doctor First

Any type of diet change needs a medical professional's approval. Schedule an appointment before starting on the Sonoma Diet. Your doctor can also help you determine the weight goal that will guide you as you follow the diet.

combines the Mediterranean secret of heart-protective eating with the Sonoman emphasis on healthy mealtime pleasure—and puts them both in a weight loss plan that works.

The result is a triple reward you may have never expected to get from a weight-loss diet: on the Sonoma Diet, you will lose weight and gain health while you enjoy your meals more than ever before.

THE NEXT STEP DIET

One subject inevitably comes up when the Sonoma Diet is introduced: Is it low-carbohydrate or low-fat?

The short answer is "neither." But the most accurate answer may be this: "The question is irrelevant."

The very fact that it arises is a sign of the times. These days popular wisdom holds that weight loss depends on drastically upsetting the carbohydrate/fat/protein balance. So diets swing like a pendulum from low-fat to low-carb.

That leaves a lot of diet dropouts feeling unsatisfied and confused. The low-fat diets tell us that food should taste dull and leave us hungry. The low-carb diets deny us our daily bread and turn vegetables and fruits into the enemy. Either way, losing weight becomes an exercise in self-denial.

Sound familiar?

The Sonoma Diet is the "next step" diet. It has nothing to do with low-carb or high-carb. It has nothing to do with low-fat or high-fat. The food choices and portion control built into the diet are calculated for the best balance of protein, carbohydrates, and fats. That balance will keep you satisfied at every step of your weight-loss journey.

The "next step" recognizes that artificially low levels of dietary fat are neither pleasing nor healthy. There's even recent evidence that low-fat diets contribute to depression.

Essential Fats

Fats are absolutely essential to a healthy diet, especially when you're trying to lose weight. They add flavour to increase the pleasure of good foods. They help your body absorb nutrients, so you can get more nutritional benefit without eating more. And healthy fats, such as nuts, create a feeling of satiety at meals, so you don't leave the table feeling hungry.

Carb Benefits

"Next step" also means acknowledging that across-the-board limits on carbohydrates doom even the most dedicated dieters to failure. Low-carb is a strategy that cannot be maintained because it's unhealthy and unsatisfying.

As most people know these days, carbohydrates are the foods most directly converted in the body to energy. They're found in whole grains, vegetables, and fruits—all great foods.

The Sonoma Diet is all about . . .

BALANCE. It has nothing to do with low-carb or low-fat.

WHOLE GRAINS. You'll be eating bread and cereal from Day 1.

POWER FOODS. Generous amounts of delicious, nutrient-dense foods help you lose weight.

HEALTH. It's based on the Mediterranean diet, which has helped protect southern Europeans from heart disease and other killers for centuries.

PLEASURE. You'll slow down to savour and enjoy your meals, Sonoma style.

MOUTHWATERING RECIPES. Straight from the culinary masters of California's Sonoma County—simple, elegant, and delicious.

OLIVE OIL. This heart-healthy, nutrition-boosting, flavour-enhancing plant oil shatters the myth that dietary fat is evil.

SIMPLICITY. You won't count calories or anything else. We did all that for you.

VARIETY. You can pick and choose the foods you want each day from generous lists of meats, seafoods, fruits, vegetables, grains, and other food types.

EASY INSTRUCTIONS. Just fill your plate or bowl according to the proportions given on page 68 for Wave 1 and 79 for Waves 2 and 3.

FRESH WHOLE FOODS. The emphasis is on the sun-drenched, flavour-packed, nutrient-rich treats like the ones from Sonoma's farms and ranches.

WINE. Thank the Mediterraneans for showing us that a glass of wine at dinner enhances your heart health as well as your meal.

SATISFACTION. The meals are complete and keep you satisfied.

Carbs also include fibre. Fibre is not only essential for digestive and cardiovascular health but also a key player in the physiology of weight loss.

Clearly, you need energy, nutrients, and fibre. That's why you need proper amounts of carbohydrates.

It is illogical for a diet to severely limit a category of food that includes healthy whole grains, vegetables, and fruits. It sends a message that there's a contradiction between losing weight and reaping the health benefits of high-fibre, nutrient-rich foods. It's a false message. Dieters sense that intuitively, which is another reason there are so many low-carb dropouts.

EATING: The Sonoma Diet Way
What's a "dietary fat"? It could be animal fat such as the marble in prime rib, a dairy fat such as butter, the "trans fats" in margarine, plant oils, the oils in fish, or the fat in seeds and nuts. You will not be given the unrealistic and unhealthy instruction to severely limit your consumption of all of those fats. Instead you'll be moderating and in some cases eliminating as much as possible of the first three, mostly because of their proven harm to your overall health.

On the Sonoma Diet, you will eat bread and cereals from the very first day. You'll have your fill of meat and fish, of course, but you'll also be encouraged to enjoy a variety of tastily prepared vegetables from Day 1.

After a 10-day transition period, fruits will be part of your diet as well. In fact, several fruits are considered the Sonoma Diet "Power Foods," meaning they'll be a high-priority food choice.

We Eat Foods, Not Categories

If there's one underlying philosophy to the "next step" diet approach, it is this: Worrying about how much carbohydrate or dietary fat you're consuming is a distraction. Keeping track of nutritional categories such as "carbohydrate," "protein," or "dietary fat" just isn't the way normal folks go about planning their meals. And that's true whether you need to lose weight or not.

Eating too many carbohydrates, especially refined ones—along with eating too much of everything—is a definite contributor to being overweight. Carbohydrates are the most likely to be over-consumed because of their effect on blood sugar metabolism (which we'll get into later).

But the solution is not to compensate for too much carbohydrate (or fat) with too little. After some initial success, your body will rebel at the carb deprivation. So will your mind. You run the risk of becoming another low-carb (or low-fat) diet dropout. You're even a candidate for the infamous rebound effect, where you end up weighing more than when you started the restrictive diet.

Rebounding is much less likely with the Sonoma Diet. As mentioned, the food guidelines and meal plans already have the ideally balanced carb/protein/fat ratio built into them. The calculations are calibrated to the three stages, or "waves," of your weight-loss programme. The amounts are set at the levels most conducive to losing weight without creating an artificial shortage of carbs or anything else that leaves you feeling deprived.

You'll never have to think about whether you're eating too many or too few carbohydrates. In fact, after this chapter you'll see the word "carb" only occasionally in the rest of this book. Instead, you can turn your attention to the soul of the Sonoma Diet— enjoying the best-tasting and healthiest foods in amounts and combinations that will get you to your target body weight quickly, safely, and permanently.

In other words, the choices you'll be making are not between scientific categories such as carbohydrate, protein, and dietary fat but involve choosing the healthiest, nutrient-rich foods within those categories.

You'll be eating controlled amounts of healthy fats. This is especially true for olive oil, an amazingly heart-healthy and flavourful oil that's a cornerstone of the Sonoma Diet. Olive oil is not a fat that you are reluctantly "allowed" to eat. Instead, you are actively encouraged to include it with your meals as a key component in your weight-loss strategy.

It's the same with carbohydrates. The Sonoma Diet includes bread and cereal from the start, while other diets spurn them. But white bread and

---

What people are saying about Sonoma ...

"This diet is amazing! I love the fact there is no counting involved and it's really easy to follow. Yeah, the first 10 days are tough, but after that, it gets a lot easier. The food is great, you don't have to give up carbs, and I don't feel hungry! My husband, who claims to not be following the diet very closely, has lost 15 lb. We're cooking and eating a lot healthier and feeling great! It's really changed the way we eat and how we'll continue to eat. I would recommend this diet to my family and friends."
Bethany, age 26, weight loss to date: 10 lb

other foods made from refined white flour (many crackers, pasta, and cereals) will indeed be virtually eliminated, for reasons we'll explain beginning on page 44. At the same time, though, you will be urged to enjoy healthy amounts of those same breads, crackers, pastas, and cereals if they're made from whole, unrefined versions of grains, such as wheat, oats, rye, and barley.

White bread and whole grain bread are both considered carbohydrates. But they're not the same. The first will sabotage your weight-loss programme faster than any other food except sugar. The second, on the other hand, is a fibre-rich, nutrient-loaded pleasure food that is so beneficial for your weight-loss goals you'll find it listed with olive oil among the "Power Foods" in the next chapter.

Add the starring role of fruits and vegetables and you get a pretty good idea that the Sonoma Diet isn't about low-carb or low-fat. It's about eating controlled but satisfying amounts of healthy, great-tasting foods, regardless of their category.

Let's Get Real

Before these words reached your eyes, the Sonoma Diet was conceived, designed, tested, adjusted, and re-tested by experts to ensure maximum efficacy for its twin goals of weight loss and improved health and vitality. The

---

EATING: The Sonoma Diet Way

The list of protein choices includes a wonderful variety of fish, shellfish, lean meat, poultry, soya, and eggs. We ask you to fill a certain percentage of your plate with something from the protein list at most meals. Though we make suggestions and encourage variety, we don't insist on any particular protein to fulfil that requirement.

So if you like, you can eat red meat seven days a week—as long as it's lean! Conversely, you may choose never to eat meat and fill your protein requirement by eating fish or eggs, or even going with soya or bean dishes. This "you make the call" method is the only realistic approach to a weight-loss plan. Dedicated carnivores can no more be expected to do without meat than vegetarians can be expected to eat it.

---

result is a proven plan that will help you lose weight—quickly at first and then steadily until you reach your goal.

But no diet will work if you can't stay with it. And you won't stay with any diet that's too complicated, too challenging, or too boring. That's why we had volunteers who struggle with the same weight issues you do test the Sonoma Diet. We knew it wasn't enough for a diet to be scientifically sound. It has to work in the real world.

Let's face it. Most of us already have enough to worry about. We have jobs to do, spouses to keep happy, children to raise, a home to maintain, and a life to live. The last thing we need is a demanding food regimen that turns mealtime into a stress-filled ordeal of complicated rules, calorie counting, and "diet dishes" that nobody likes.

The Sonoma Diet is none of those things. We made sure everything about this diet is enjoyable, simple, and satisfying. Most of all, we kept it realistic.

You don't need to be an amateur nutritionist to follow this diet. We've done all the thinking for you. You won't count carbs, and you won't count calories. We've already counted them. All you have to do is choose foods from long lists of options and put them on your plate in the proportions we give you.

Yes, you'll need to prepare most of the meals. But we make that easy too. The recipes we provide are not only quick and simple to follow, they're also based on the Sonoma cuisine that's among the most praised (and healthiest) in the world. You'll be amazed at how great a cook you've become.

No matter where you live, you can lose weight following the Sonoma Diet. We've made sure that the ingredients are affordable and easy to find. You'll do best on the diet if you try foods and dishes from the lists that are new to you. Variety is your ally. But there's nothing on the lists that isn't readily available at your local farmer's market or supermarket.

You will not be asked to change your meal habits. No switching from three squares to a five-a-day plan. No restrictions on what time you eat dinner or breakfast or anything else. All we ask is that you sit down, take your time, and enjoy your meals. Have a glass of wine with one of them if you like. Let mealtime be stress-reduction time. That's the Sonoma way.

Snacks are fine on the Sonoma Diet. If a snack helps keep you from feeling hungry, by all means have one. You can't eat just anything between meals, of course. Like everything else on the diet, you need to snack on the right amount of the right things. We tell you what those are. Look for some suggestions on pages 73 and 88. More options are listed with the meal plans beginning on page 160.

There's another reality-based touch that you'll appreciate. The Sonoma Diet asks you to abandon your bad eating habits, but not your personal eating habits. The variety on the food lists and the flexibility in choices make sure you can eat the way you always have. You'll eat less, you'll eat healthier, and you'll eat slower. But you'll still choose the foods you like best.

Simple for Busy Lives

You'll find the Sonoma Diet amazingly easy to follow.

The three basic factors that determine your weight loss are food selection (what you eat), food combination (what your meals consist of), and portion control (how much you eat). The unique "plate-and-bowl" concept you'll be using makes each of those a very simple proposition. At the same time, so much variety is offered that you may never repeat the same meal twice.

What people are saying about Sonoma ...

"I have been very happy with my success on the Sonoma Diet. I have been surprised at how easily I've been able to adapt the diet to my active lifestyle. Best of all, I haven't been hungry!"
Jaimie, age 27, weight loss to date: 20.5 lb

Food selection couldn't be simpler. It's merely a matter of lists. For example, every grain that is okay to eat is listed under "Sonoma Grains." Every acceptable fat appears on the list "Sonoma Fats." There are also lists of approved choices in the following categories: proteins (meats, fish, beans, etc.), dairy, fruits, vegetables, flavour boosters, and beverages.

Your fruit and vegetable options are divided into levels, or "tiers." Tiering simply recognizes that some foods in a category are more conducive to weight loss than others. Tier 1 vegetables, for example, may be enjoyed often in all stages of the diet. These include asparagus, aubergines, spinach, and tomatoes, among others. Vegetables from Tier 2 (such as artichokes and carrots) and Tier 3 (including sweetcorn and sugar snap peas) will be eaten more sparingly—and not at all during the initial wave of the diet. A similar tiering system applies to fruit.

When the diet instructions call for a certain amount of proteins or grains or anything else in a meal, all you have to do is consult the appropriate list and choose what you're in the mood for that day.

On the other side of the coin, there are two lists of foods that you should not eat. The first is a more restrictive list of foods to be avoided only during the early waves of your diet. The other lists foods to be shunned throughout the diet, and even after. These are the foods that will sabotage your weight-loss progress and raise your risk of heart disease and other illnesses. You'll see that they're mostly saturated fats, sugar, and refined flour products such as white bread, cakes, and biscuits.

Redefining the (American) Plate (and Bowl)

How much do you eat at each meal? That's where the plate-and-bowl concept comes in. This concept brings the most recent nutrition science to your plate. It redefines the common American plate, heavily criticized for its super-sized portions, calories, and fat. The emphasis is a shift in focus, for more vegetables and grains to play centre stage in the company of lean meats. You'll be using an 18-cm/7-inch plate or a 450 ml/¾ pint bowl for your breakfast and a 23-cm/9-inch plate for your lunch and dinner. The diet instructions (which are explained and illustrated beginning on page 61 for Wave 1 and page 77 for Wave 2) will tell you how to fill those plates and bowl.

For example, a typical Wave 1 dinner will call for filling your 23-cm/9-inch plate with 30% protein, 20% grains, and 50% Tier 1 vegetables. So you might want to fill half your plate with a raw spinach and vegetable salad. A salmon fillet can fill the 30% protein segment and wild rice (never white rice) the rest.

You'll welcome this concept as a lot easier than counting grams or ounces. Because the plates are set in size, the portion control is automatic. You don't measure; you just fill. And because we tell you the amount of each food type that goes on the plate, you're assured of getting the best combination for healthy weight loss. This is a style of eating that will make you more aware of what's on your plate, long after you reach your target body weight.

In addition to the fat found naturally in your food (in meats, salad dressings, and so on), you'll choose additional fats to add flavour to your food and keep you full. Your daily fat allotment is measured in teaspoons of plant oil or individual nuts, so they won't appear as percentages on your plate diagram. Your beverages and flavour boosters don't need to be measured at all—they're limitless.

Losing Weight in Waves

The way you'll feel at the beginning of your diet is not how you'll feel as the weeks pass by. This is good news, because you'll feel better. The diet gets easier as time passes, not harder. There are lots of reasons for this. Two stand out.

One is that you'll be enjoying your meals more than you did before you started the diet. Remember, the recipes you'll use are inspired by Sonoma cuisine—a style of cooking that's as noted for its full, robust flavours as it is for its healthy goodness.

The other is that somewhere around 10 days into the diet, perhaps earlier, you'll realize that the portions determined by the Sonoma Diet plate-and-bowl concept are big enough to satisfy you at every meal. You'll wonder how you managed to eat those huge servings you helped yourself to before.

For these reasons, we've divided your diet into three distinct "waves." Wave 1 lasts the first 10 days. It's during this period that you'll be overcoming your habit of consuming large amounts of sugars, refined flour products, and other fast-absorbing foods that most likely led to your weight concerns in the first place.

The list of restricted foods is longer in Wave 1. Fruits, because of their natural sugar content, are on hold for these 10 days. But you'll still have full, rich meals—with whole grain bread or cereal, meat or fish, and plenty of vegetables.

In Wave 1, you're naturally recalibrating the body and turning around bad eating habits a lifetime in the making. This challenge comes right at the beginning, when your enthusiasm and confidence are in high gear. You'll be thrilled with the results, since this is the period of fastest weight loss. And right when you're fully adjusted to your new healthy eating habits, your portions and choices increase.

Now you're in Wave 2. This is the main leg of the diet, where you'll stay until you reach your target weight. Weight loss is not as quick as it was in the first wave, but it comes steadily. During this wave you'll continue cultivating the Sonoma approach to eating, where each meal is savoured slowly with an emphasis on health and pleasure.

For Waves 1 and 2, we provide you with a daily meal guide that gives precise dishes (with recipes) that match the instructions for filling your plate or bowl with the right balance, variety, and combinations of food. This meal guide will tell you exactly what to eat for breakfast, lunch, and dinner for each of the 10 days in Wave 1 and for 14-day cycles in Wave 2.

For example, in Wave 1, your lunch or dinner plate must be filled with 30% protein, 20% grains, and 50% Tier 1 vegetables. On each day of Wave 1, we will provide you with a different lunch or dinner meal that follows those proportions precisely.

These meal guides make your meal planning even easier, since all you have to do for any meal is prepare what we tell you to. But it's optional. As long as you follow the plate-filling instructions and food lists, you can choose whatever you want. Specific instructions or freedom of choice? It's up to you.

Wave 3 starts the day you reach your target weight. Since congratulations will be in order, your wine choice for the day just might be a bit of the bubbly. Now it's time to convert your new appreciation of healthy eating from a weight-loss diet into a lifestyle.

By Wave 3, you'll know what works best for you. Your portion control and food choices will come naturally, and you won't need percentage instructions. Unlimited fruits and vegetables are yours to enjoy. You'll also want to give yourself a special treat now and then. If at any point you find your weight starting to creep up, just pull out those plates and bowls and start back on Wave 2.

The Top Ten Sonoma Diet Power Foods

"What are we NOT having for dinner tonight?" Probably not a question that you ask or hear. Human beings don't think that way about food. We look forward to what we're going to enjoy, not to what we're going to shun. We eat positively, not negatively.

Most popular diets, however, go about things in just the opposite fashion. With their strict prohibitions regarding fats, carbs, and other essentials, these diets border on cruelty. You enter into a diet like that with clenched fists and gritted teeth, trying to summon the willpower to somehow "make it through" long months of imposed austerity.

No wonder so many end up rebounding to a higher weight than they started with. We don't like deprivation. Sooner or later we're going to rebel.

Some restrictions, of course, make sense. You aren't going to lose weight by eating all the banana cream pie and nacho platters you can get your hands on. But deprivation cannot be the central focus of a successful diet—moderation, balance, and smart choices are the keys to success.

Heart-Healthy Whole Foods

The central focus of the Sonoma Diet is the abundant variety of healthy and delicious, fresh whole foods you'll be having every day. You'll lose weight not by avoiding food but by enjoying appropriate amounts of the best foods.

When people enjoy a typical meal from the Sonoma Diet, such as grilled seasoned chicken, brown rice, steamed broccoli seasoned with tarragon and oregano, and strawberries, accompanied by a glass of Pinot Noir, they're not thinking about the potato crisps and cream cheese dip they could have had instead. They're too busy savouring the flavourful meal in front of them to worry about what's not there.

When you sit down for that same meal (perfect for Wave 2, by the way), you'll feel the same way. The fact that the feast in front of you will add to your health and subtract from your weight is almost like a bonus. The last thing in the world you should feel like when you're enjoying a meal is that you're "on a diet."

Mediterranean Eating

The Sonoma Diet works because we've inherited from our Mediterranean friends a lengthy roster of delicious foods that offer exceptional nutritional value but relatively few calories. What's more, many of them are proven protective against heart disease and other serious illnesses. They're the secret to the Mediterranean diet.

Top Ten Power Foods

Almonds	Olive Oil
Peppers	Spinach
Blueberries	Strawberries
Broccoli	Tomatoes
Grapes	Whole Grains

In scientific jargon, these foods are notable for their "nutrient richness." More casually put, they're the ones that offer the most nutritional bang for the calorie buck. These foods are the backbone of the Sonoma Diet and a big reason why health and weight loss go hand in hand.

It gets even better. Some nutrient-rich foods pack more nutrients than others, while some have other special qualities that give them an honoured place on your plate. We call these power foods. There are plenty of them, but we've selected the Top Ten Power Foods for you to focus on as you plan your meals.

Before we jump into Wave 1, let's get to know the Top Ten Power Foods. After all, you'll be eating them regularly for the rest of your life. And they'll be your best friends and closest allies as you march towards your target weight.

First, though, let's take a look at what puts the power in power foods.

The Power of Nutrients

Here's a question you may not have thought about: Why do we eat?

If you answered, "Because we're hungry," go to the back of the room.

If you answered, "To give our bodies energy and building material," you found the right answer. But it's incomplete.

We also eat to provide our bodies with certain chemical substances that act in beneficial ways. These are nutrients. More specifically, they are "essential" nutrients, so-called because they aren't manufactured in the body itself. They must come from food.

Your cells use these nutrients to carry out their functions properly. When they get enough of the nutrients they need, you are more likely to be healthy. When they get those nutrients in low-calorie packages, you are more likely to get to your best weight. That's the value of power foods.

Phytonutrients

At the top of the Sonoma Diet power foods list are plant foods, whose power is mostly attributed to their phytonutrients ("phyto" is Greek for plant). Vitamins and minerals play a big role, of course. But the discovery in recent decades of a huge variety of almost-magical plant chemicals has confirmed what every grandmother has known for centuries—that vegetables, fruits, and grains are bursting with health and goodness.

Phytochemicals are primarily responsible for the unique colours, flavours, and textures of fruits and vegetables. There are hundreds, perhaps thousands, of phytochemicals with an overwhelming vocabulary of hard-to-pronounce names and ways in which they provide health benefits. But two broad categories of phytochemicals are worth knowing: flavonoids and carotenoids. These nutrient types are responsible not only for the distinctive colouring of most of the Top Ten Power Foods but also for their extensive health benefits.

Antioxidants

Flavonoids, carotenoids, and other phytochemicals in the power foods work in lots of ways, but one stands out—their antioxidant action.

Antioxidants have got plenty of attention in the last decade, and it's all deserved. Antioxidants protect the body from potentially harmful substances, known as free radicals. Free radicals travel through the body causing damage to cells. This damage leads to a build-up of cholesterol in the arteries and may cause heart disease, certain forms of cancer, diabetes, cataracts, arthritis, and perhaps even Alzheimer's disease.

One last thing about phytonutrients. Though some (such as lycopene and beta-carotene) play starring roles, they almost always work together with vitamins and minerals. That means it's important to eat a variety of whole foods in various combinations.

You'll find that easy to do with all ten of the top power foods that follow.

ALMONDS: A MIGHTY NUT

You'll find almonds in a surprising number of dishes in Sonoma restaurants and homes. In the United States, they're grown exclusively in California. Their sweet taste is one reason they're so popular. As with so many of the Sonoma Diet foods, the marriage of pleasure and health in almonds is a solid one.

Full of Health Benefits

It may surprise you that a food relatively high in calories such as almonds makes the list of power foods. The fact is all calories, especially fat calories, are not created equal. The fat in almonds is primarily heart-healthy monounsaturated fat, the same type found in olives, olive oil, avocados, and other nuts. There is a growing consensus among the medical community that almonds decrease the risk for heart disease. Recent medical studies found that eating 25 g/1 oz of almonds daily (about a handful), as part of a healthy lifestyle, reduces LDL cholesterol (the bad stuff) and thereby reduces your overall heart disease risk. Other studies have shown that almonds are protective against cancer and diabetes as well. And eating almonds on a regular basis may decrease other risk factors in the blood that are related to artery-damaging inflammation. An exciting discovery in these studies was that the addition of the extra daily calories from almonds did not lead to any weight gain in the participants.

SHOPPING: The Sonoma Diet Way
Choose plain almonds, not sugar- or salt-coated ones. To bring out the flavour at home, toast them for a few minutes in a warm oven.

Could there be some nutrients in almonds that actually help you lose weight? The answer appears to be yes! One explanation may be that the fat contained in almonds is not completely absorbed into the body. This is related to the fibrous make-up of almonds. The other explanation is that almonds provide just the right combination of nutrients such as protein, fat, fibre, vitamins, and minerals to curb hunger.

Nutrient Rich

Almonds stand out as especially rich in calcium—in fact, they're one of the best non-dairy calcium sources. They also deliver plenty of protein, copper, zinc, potassium, magnesium, and B vitamins.

And like all the other power foods, almonds supply antioxidant nutrients, most notably in this case vitamin E.

Almonds are a classic example of the positive benefits of power foods that go beyond the specific nutrients they supply. Focusing on eating good foods, such as almonds, is a more direct route to your target weight than concentrating only on avoiding "bad" foods. A typical "low-fat" diet might discourage eating almonds. That's counterproductive. Almonds, in proper amounts, can help you avoid eating problem fats. A revealing 2004 study published in a British medical journal illustrated this. About 80 men and women were told to eat 25 g / 1 oz of almonds every day but were given no other diet instructions. After six months, on their own, the almond eaters had noticeably cut down on the amount of harmful saturated fats and trans-fatty acids they were eating.

In other words, by eating a smart fat—almonds—they automatically avoided problem fats. That's exactly what you'll be doing.

PEPPERS:
RINGING IN THE NUTRIENTS

How can such a seemingly lightweight vegetable be bursting with nutrition? Well, that's what makes peppers such a solid Sonoma power food—lots of health-imparting nutrients and a miniscule amount of calories (about 35).

They're also a classic Mediterranean vegetable—think stuffed peppers, or raw pepper strips in a brightly coloured spring salad. Brought to southern Europe from the New World by the Spanish in the 16th century, peppers grow anywhere that's not too cold. That includes Sonoma, where locally grown versions are sold fresh at farmers' markets.

The Sonoma Diet Food Tip:

Taste peppers in a variety of colours and notice the subtle flavour differences. All the colours are loaded with nutrients, so you can't go wrong. And they're healthy and tasty raw or cooked.

The power of peppers is right there in the colours. Green, purple, red, yellow, and orange are all phytonutrient-rich peppers. But the nature of some of the nutrients changes with the colour. Not that it matters, because the heart-healthy, cancer-preventive, sight-saving benefits abound with any hue.

Heart Protection

What all those coloured peppers have in common are generous natural doses of the antioxidant vitamins A and C. These two vitamins protect against heart disease by discouraging LDL in the bloodstream from the oxidation process that makes the bad cholesterol worse. Two other vitamins abundant in peppers—B_6 and folic acid—help out by lowering levels of a heart-disease-related protein called homocysteine.

Cancer Fighting

While peppers of all colours are rich in antioxidant carotenoids, the red ones pack a bonus in the form of lycopene. This is a powerful antioxidant that gives tomatoes and red peppers their colour. Its specialty is cancer fighting. The evidence is clear that a daily dose of lycopene, along with the vitamins and beta-carotene (another carotenoid) found in peppers, reduces your risk of colon, cervix, bladder, pancreas, and prostate cancers.

Peppers' potent combination of carotenoids and antioxidant vitamins also appears to offer protection against lung disease and lung cancer. Here, too, red and orange peppers may provide an extra boost because of a special carotenoid called beta-cryptoxanthin, which is found in other orange foods as well—from pumpkin to papaya.

Vision Preservation

There's also evidence that the antioxidants in peppers help stave off age-related vision problems, such as cataracts. Once again, red peppers may be the best choice for your eyes, because they alone contain some special nutrients thought to protect against macular degeneration, a common cause of vision loss.

The beauty of peppers is their built-in variety. You'll find all kinds of ways to enjoy peppers as you progress through your diet. And you'll start right in on them at Wave 1.

BLUEBERRIES: AN EVERYDAY SPECIAL TREAT

Everybody loves blueberries, but how often do people eat them? Some never do. Others only think about blueberries that are baked in muffins. Their loss. Blueberries are an especially potent power food.

If you've always thought of blueberries as a rare special treat, think of them now as a common special treat. Work them into your meal planning as soon as you hit Wave 2 of the diet. Yes,

EATING: The Sonoma Diet Way

In Sonoma fresh sweet blueberries dropped into whole grain cereals, topped with fat-free yogurt, or just popped into your mouth one by one, are part of the healthy lifestyle. It's not uncommon for folks there to pick ripe blueberries right off the bush to take home to eat.

they're usually a tad pricier than most of the Sonoma Diet foods, but you'll be alternating them with more than a dozen other Tier 2 fruits, including several other berry types.

Give blueberries some priority, though. They're worth the extra pennies. There's a good reason why they're high on the power food list.

The Power of Antioxidants

The magic of blueberries comes from the astonishing amounts of antioxidants they contain. The U.S. Department of Agriculture recently conducted a sort of antioxidant census and among fruits, blueberries led the league. Based on what we currently know, only one food on the planet (red kidney beans) offers more antioxidants per serving than blueberries.

Many of those antioxidants are the same flavonoids responsible for the heart-strengthening benefits of grapes and wine. That includes resveratrol, one of the true Hall of Fame nutrients on the Sonoma Diet team, thanks to its well-documented heart-protecting abilities. But blueberries, it turns out, pack even more resveratrol than wine.

Not surprisingly, that wine-like antioxidant action puts blueberries among the elite of Sonoma-style heart-healthy foods. But recent research has uncovered another amazing benefit. Eating blueberries regularly may slow down, and perhaps even reverse, the memory decline that comes with ageing. That same brain-saving ability is also found in strawberries and spinach—two other power foods included in the Sonoma Diet.

Blueberries reduce your risk of a whole slew of illnesses, including certain types of cancer, vision loss, and digestive disorders. One other protective effect, however, stands out.

You probably know about cranberries' ability to fend off urinary tract infections. Blueberries contain the same bacteria-inhibiting phytonutrients as cranberries. Investigators still need to find direct evidence that blueberries work against urinary tract infections as effectively as cranberries. In the meantime, though, the probability that they do help gives you one more reason to indulge often in these sweet treats.

BROCCOLI: A GOURMET POWER FOOD

Broccoli is about as Mediterranean as a vegetable can be. It began in Italy, then the Romans spread it through Europe, and immigrants took it to America. Raw or cooked, it's a super player in the Sonoma Diet, something for you to eat in virtually unlimited amounts for the rest of your life.

Vitamin C and Calcium

You probably don't need convincing when it comes to broccoli's benefits. Its reputation as one of the world's healthiest foods is established. But did you know that broccoli is one of the best sources for calcium and vitamin C?

Consider this. There's as much vitamin C in a serving of broccoli (that's 50 g/2 oz in the Sonoma Diet) as in an orange. But an orange will set you back 60 to 70 calories—not a huge amount, but considerably more than the 20 or so in a serving of broccoli. That's why broccoli is a power food.

Same goes for calcium. A 50 g/2 oz serving of broccoli delivers about 40 milligrams of calcium—a decent amount. Sure, you'll get more than that in 225 ml/8 fl oz of milk, but you'll also get 85 to 150 calories, depending on what kind of milk you're drinking. And milk—even skimmed milk—has some saturated fat. Broccoli has zero fat of any kind. That's right. None.

COOKING: The Sonoma Diet Way

Don't overcook your broccoli into a soggy, nutrient-depleted mush. Use the Sonoma Diet recipes beginning on page 166. Take advantage of the huge selection of herbs, spices, and other flavour enhancers you can use at any phase of the Sonoma Diet. Or eat broccoli raw. You can enjoy fresh broccoli just like you'd enjoy carrots. Chomp away. You're doing your health and your body weight a favour.

Cancer Fighter

Beyond its role as a rich source of vitamin C and calcium, broccoli is a deluxe detoxifier. It's the Mr Clean of vegetables, clearing away potentially carcinogenic toxins and even inhibiting tumour growth. That makes broccoli a strong cancer fighter. Is there a nobler effort a power food can make?

Interestingly, the big anti-cancer gun in broccoli's phytonutrient arsenal is a detoxifier called sulphorophane. As the name hints, this is the substance responsible for the sulphur-like smell of broccoli as it cooks. That's turned off many a kid and former president to this gift of nature.

But there's no sulphurish taste at all to broccoli. Properly cooking broccoli, such as lightly steaming it, enhances its flavour even more. Broccoli's a true gourmet vegetable as well as a cancer fighter and heart protector.

GRAPES: FRUIT OF THE GODS

The Greeks and Romans considered grapes a gift from the gods. And why not? There's something miraculous about a gnarly black vine creating generous clusters of bright pearls of fruit, each bursting with pure goodness.

These ancient southern Europeans appreciated the health-imparting power of grapes themselves. But they positively worshipped the fruit's capacity to convert itself into that most sensuous of nectars—fine wine.

The Greeks and Romans bequeathed their love of grapes and wine to their modern southern European successors, who turned both into cornerstones of the Mediterranean diet.

Grapes are equally revered in today's Sonoma. There the hillsides are covered with vineyards, their ripening fruit gleaming green and purple in the pre-harvest sun. The Sonoma Diet is indebted to this important part of the Sonoma economy.

Heart Protection

What's wonderful about grapes as a power food is that they deliver virtually all of the nutrients that wine does. That means you'll still reap most of the heart-protective and weight-loss benefits of grapes' abundant phytonutrients even if you cannot (or choose not to) drink a daily glass of wine.

Grapes and wine are a big reason modern researchers got curious about the Mediterranean diet in the first place. Why, they asked, did southern Europeans suffer so few heart attacks even as they ate so richly? A big reason, we know now, is the special potency of the heart-protective nutrients in the grapes and wine they consume so liberally.

The phytonutrients in grapes work to keep your entire cardiovascular system healthy in the usual way. That is, they protect the blood vessels and heart muscle itself from tissue damage by free radicals and the "rusting" they can cause.

It would take an organic chemistry textbook to describe the myriad flavonoids that make grapes such a heart-healthy food. But you've already met the most important one — resveratrol, the same wonder nutrient that powers blueberries.

While there's actually more resveratrol in blueberries than in grapes, the supporting cast in grapes is unbeatable. Because the flavonoids and other antioxidant nutrients work together like a philharmonic orchestra, grapes have achieved elite power-food status.

Whole Food Benefits

They also make a great argument for the whole-foods approach to weight loss. Studies abound confirming the heart-protecting benefits of eating grapes and drinking wine. But the evidence for resveratrol acting alone in supplement form is much skimpier.

Red or purple grapes are richer in flavonoids than the white or green varieties, but we're not going to hold you to that. Grapes of any colour are power foods.

You won't, however, be able to eat grapes without limits until you reach your weight goal. Their high sugar content puts them on the Tier 2 list, meaning you can enjoy 50 g/2 oz of grapes a day starting with Wave 2.

You'll probably want to alternate them with other Tier 2 fruits, but give them priority. Grapes are the very symbol of Sonoma's healthy way of life.

OLIVE OIL: A WEIGHT-LOSS BLESSING

In Sonoma County each year, there's a special festival called the Blessing of the Olives. That's how central olive trees and the foods they yield are to the economy and the eating habits of the region.

Olive oil, the most treasured gift of these blessed trees, is just as central to the Sonoma Diet. There's probably no food choice you'll make that does more for your health and weight-loss efforts than olive oil.

SHOPPING: The Sonoma Diet Way
Always buy extra-virgin olive oil. "Extra-virgin" simply means that the oil comes from the first pressing of the olives and therefore retains the most beneficial nutrients. It also has by far the most delicate and pleasing taste.

Which is good news for your taste buds, because no other vegetable oil comes close to olive oil's rich and pleasing flavour. It's at the heart of Mediterranean cuisine's appeal. A dish prepared with olive oil almost seems to announce to anyone who smells or tastes it, "I'm special."

Healthy Fat

The research is clear as can be that a major reason for southern Europeans' low rate of heart disease is their liberal use of olive oil as their main source of dietary fat. By adopting olive oil in the same way, you'll get the same benefits. And because you'll learn to enjoy olive oil in healthy amounts in place of the harmful fats you may be used to, you will lose weight.

To appreciate olive oil as a power food, banish from your mind the notion that it's the "least bad" fat. It is a heart-healthy food that is good for you. You need dietary fat to lose weight, but you need the right kind. Olive oil is one of the best. Choose extra-virgin olive oil and you'll also enhance the flavours of your food.

Put simply, the kind of fat that olive oil is mostly made of (monounsaturated fat) actually lowers your levels of the bad LDL cholesterol as well as blood fats called triglycerides. The fats you'll be avoiding (saturated fat) raise those levels. That right there qualifies olive oil as a power food par excellence.

COOKING: The Sonoma Diet Way

A big advantage you'll get from using olive oil regularly is its special ability to interact with other foods. Try olive oil as a dressing over a spinach salad, for example. It not only improves the flavour by toning down the subtle bitterness of the leaves; it also boosts the action of all those beneficial phytonutrients in spinach.

A Wealth of Antioxidants

But there's more. Unique among vegetable oils, olive oil—particularly extra-virgin olive oil—is rich in the same family of antioxidant phytonutrients that make all the other power foods on the Top Ten list so effective in preventing heart disease. The same phenols that make olive oil taste so good also make up its main category of antioxidants. Olive oil also contains carotenoids (like beta-carotene) and vitamin E.

In addition, olive oil reduces two other heart disease risks—high blood pressure and inflammation.

SPINACH: FULL OF SURPRISES

This is the quintessential "green leafy vegetable" so often recommended for overall health. In fact that's what spinach basically is—big green leaves (though the stems are great too). What's in those leaves borders on the miraculous.

Calorie for calorie, spinach is a valuable power food. The nutritional benefits are so abundant—and the calories so negligible—you can eat virtually all you want of this amazing plant. Like tomatoes, broccoli, and peppers, spinach is a Tier 1 vegetable that you can eat plenty of from the first day of your diet, and in unlimited amounts once you reach Wave 2.

COOKING: The Sonoma Diet Way

Raw and cooked spinach are almost like two different foods, their taste and presentation are so different. When cooking spinach, try lightly steaming it to preserve the majority of its phytonutrients. Raw, however, in the form of a tasty spinach salad, is best. Drizzle on extra-virgin olive oil, add some toasted nuts, or check out the dressings in the recipe section. No need to be too picky, though. However you like it, spinach is an all-star power food you'll be enjoying a lot.

Nutrient Rich

Spinach is full of pleasant surprises. It's a natural source of iron, making it a low-calorie source of iron that's so important to pregnant, lactating, or menstruating women. And like broccoli and almonds, it's a rich non-dairy source of calcium. The combination of calcium and vitamin K (which spinach also delivers in abundance) promotes bone health and helps prevent osteoporosis.

Keep in mind that along with blueberries and strawberries, the flavonoids in spinach are thought to slow cognitive decline, meaning they may prevent the memory loss that often accompanies ageing. Spinach is also rich in lutein, a carotenoid that a growing body of research has linked to eye health and a reduced risk of age-related vision problems.

Like most Mediterranean power foods, spinach provides a generous and varied supply of antioxidant nutrients that fight heart disease by discouraging dangerous oxidation of existing blood cholesterol. But it also protects your heart in lots of other ways, making it stand out among heart-healthy food.

For example, spinach is especially rich in folate, a B vitamin that reduces the amount of a harmful protein in your body called homocysteine. One of the more important recent findings about heart health in recent years is the connection between high homocysteine levels and your risk for a heart attack or stroke.

Another key recent discovery is the role of inflammation in heart disease. Spinach has well-known anti-inflammatory properties, so it's possible it protects your heart that way. (It certainly helps prevent inflammatory conditions such as arthritis and asthma.) There's also recent evidence that the protein in spinach contains components that help you avoid high blood pressure, a top risk factor for serious heart problems.

STRAWBERRIES: THE PLEASURE PRINCIPLE

Wash and slice 70 g/2½ oz of fresh strawberries, and you're looking at maybe 25 calories, 30 max. You're also looking at a first-rate power food that not only delivers the fibre, vitamins, and minerals you expect from a fruit but also a generous dose of especially beneficial phytochemicals. That combination makes strawberries a surprisingly potent health booster for your heart, joints, and even your mind.

COOKING: The Sonoma Diet Way

Buying organic produce is a personal choice but is recommended with strawberries, because commercial growers often use strong pesticides. Organic or not, wash your strawberries well before you eat them.

Delicious Health

If you're like most people, you probably don't think of strawberries as "health food." They taste too good, for one thing. And they're usually associated with over-sugared jams and jellies, not to mention saturated-fat-packed ice cream, or cakes and pies made with refined flour.

But that's just the kind of thinking you'll leave behind as you shed pounds with the Sonoma Diet. Strawberries are a pleasure to eat and a boon for your health and weight loss efforts. Once you realize there's more enjoyment in 70 g/2½ oz of fresh, ripe, nutrient-rich strawberries than in a strawberry pastry, you're well on your way to reaching your weight goal.

Beginning with Wave 2, you can treat yourself to a moderate amount of fresh strawberries every day. When you do, you're providing your body with a unique assortment of phenols (a broad category of phytonutrients). These are antioxidants, acting like rust busters to keep cells healthy and minimize the harm of cholesterol accumulating in your arteries.

Strawberries' special phenols have also been shown to reduce dangerous inflammation throughout the body, including the arteries. Their anti-inflammatory action appears to work much like aspirin. That provides even more heart protection, now that inflammation is considered such a major risk factor for heart disease.

Like blueberries and spinach, strawberries also contain special flavonoids that appear to have a brain-saving effect. Thus eating strawberries regularly may literally save your memory.

SHOPPING: The Sonoma Diet Way
Strawberries perish quickly but freeze (and thaw) well. So go ahead and buy a big sack of frozen straw-berries to last you for a week or so. Also look for straight-from-the-farm berries that were picked ripe; visit a local farmers' market or stop at a fresh fruit stand.

There's also abundant evidence indicating that eating strawberries regularly helps protect you from cancer, age-related vision impairment, and (because of their anti-inflammatory properties) rheumatoid arthritis.

TOMATOES: PRIDE OF THE KITCHEN

Picture a typical Mediterranean kitchen. You'll see lots of ripe red tomatoes, sliced fresh on a cutting board or simmering in an aromatic sauce. The same scene is common in Sonoma homes and restaurants, where vine-ripened and often homegrown tomatoes are key to the region's healthy and satisfying way of eating.

Your kitchen will look much the same from now on. Tomatoes are a top power food—nutrient-packed and great tasting, with barely 40 calories per piece. You're encouraged to eat plenty from Day 1 of your diet. And you'll find that it's easy to do. The beauty of tomatoes is their versatility.

The Power of Phytochemicals

What makes tomatoes such a strong ally in your healthy diet? Part of their power comes from their rich array of phytochemicals that work together to protect your cardiovascular system. That makes tomatoes a classic heart-healthy Mediterranean food.

Tomatoes' most powerful component is a phytonutrient called lycopene. This is the carotenoid that gives red tomatoes their bright colour. It's also one of the most-studied nutrients in the last decade. The evidence has repeatedly shown that lycopene in tomatoes reduces your risk of several cancers—including breast, cervix, prostate, pancreas, and lung cancers.

That puts tomatoes in a unique category. For most power foods, the scientific case for their heart-protective benefits is solid, while evidence for their cancer-fighting property is strong but incomplete. Not so for tomatoes. Their anti-cancer action is even more proven than their heart benefits.

Eating tomatoes, then, will help you lose weight, keep your heart healthy, and stay cancer-free as you grow older. That's the mark of a true power food.

Try tomatoes in all their many forms: fresh, canned, as a sauce, or as a paste. All forms are high in lycopene. Fresh tomatoes are best in the summer, so stock up and enjoy them at their peak. In the colder months, make your own tomato sauces and soups with canned tomatoes. Some canned tomatoes come with added flavours to make your cooking even easier.

SHOPPING: The Sonoma Diet Way

Try to buy vine-ripened tomatoes. "Vine-ripened" simply means the tomato reached full maturity before it was picked. Commercial suppliers generally harvest their tomatoes early and let them ripen in the store or on the way to it. That reduces spoilage but robs the tomatoes of much of their nutritional value and most of their naturally delicious flavour.

COOKING: The Sonoma Diet Way

Take advantage of tomatoes as a weight-loss food in all their variety—cut raw into salads, diced and sprinkled over lean meat, as a soup or stew base, bubbling in a flavourful tomato sauce, and in countless other guises. Canned tomatoes are a good option in the winter months. Unlike some power foods, tomatoes lose little of their nutritional potency when cooked. The research even tells us that tomatoes' cancer-preventing properties are more active in cooked tomatoes than in raw ones. Tomato purée and sauce, for example, are excellent sources of lycopene.

WHOLE GRAINS:
YOUR SECRET OF SUCCESS

Whole grains make for a special power food. They're not a single food but a category that includes whole grain bread, brown or wild rice, oatmeal, popcorn, and cereal, and bread or crackers made from whole grains with no white flour.

While some diets prohibit or severely limit any kind of grain or cereal, whole grains are the very heart and soul of the Sonoma Diet. The difference between eating whole grains and eating refined white-flour foods is the difference between reaching your weight goal and not reaching it.

Boost Metabolism

Making whole grains a part of your life is also one of the best things you can do to boost metabolism, smooth insulin release, and control blood sugar, not to mention lower your risk of diabetes, cancer, stroke, and heart disease. You are encouraged to enjoy whole grain bread and other whole grain foods in the amounts recommended in each Wave of the diet.

What makes a grain "whole"? Simply the fact that the nutrient-rich bran, germ, and endosperm have not been milled out of the grain kernel. When any cereal grain, such as rice or wheat, is processed into white flour, the natural fibre, vitamins, and beneficial phytonutrients are sacrificed, turning an otherwise potent source of nutrients into a collection of empty calories.

Worse, your bloodstream absorbs white flour so fast that your blood sugar levels first soar and then dive as the fat-producing insulin hormone rushes in as a response.

You'll learn in the next chapter why all that's so devastating to your health and body weight. Here we're looking at the positive side of the coin—whole grains' starring role in your weight-loss efforts.

Fibre Rich

First and foremost, whole grains deliver lots of the best kinds of fibre (while refined white flour delivers almost none). Fibre, as we'll see later, is your weight-loss and heart-health ally for its ability to slow cholesterol absorption and lower blood fat levels.

But while fibre gets most of the attention, it's the entire package that makes whole grains so important. Grains are plants, and they provide the same kind of nutrient boosts we expect from the best plant foods. That includes antioxidant phytonutrients with the same health benefits as all the other Top Ten Power Foods.

SHOPPING: The Sonoma Diet Way

Always look for "whole grain" or "whole wheat" as the first ingredient on a label of bread or pasta. Otherwise, the product could say "wheat" but not really include whole grains.

Like olive oil, whole grains are higher in calories, so you can't eat unlimited amounts and still lose weight. The plate diagrams and food lists will tell you the right amounts for each Wave.

Once you scan the list of the Sonoma Diet whole grain products, you'll quickly see that your choices are almost unlimited. Anything made with refined grains can be made with whole grains—breads, cereals, pasta, crackers, you name it. And of course wheat, oats, and rice are only the best-known grains. Your whole grain lists also include Sonoma-style treats that might be new to you, such as bulgur, quinoa, and the different varieties of whole grain rice.

A Food and Taste Tour of the Sonoma Diet

To lose weight, you have to love to eat.

If that sounds strange, consider the opposite side of the coin: traditional diet thinking maintains that to lose weight you must downplay the role of meals in your life and avoid food as much as possible.

Now, that really is a strange statement. It runs counter to every byte of behaviour information hardwired into our genes from millions of years of evolution. We know we need to eat to survive, and our happiest memories celebrate food, family, and friends. It's natural to resist any advice to the contrary.

If you've tried to lose weight before, you probably sensed intuitively that such an anti-food approach would be a problem. It's hard to defeat an "enemy" that you love.

The Sonoma Diet stresses enjoying food, not avoiding it. The secret, of course, is enjoying the right foods in the right amounts. That's the only healthy way to lose weight.

You will be choosing from a large variety of foods and recipes that have been shown to have the strongest of health benefits. By "health benefits" we mean that these foods make you feel better, increase your energy and vitality, and help protect you from killer diseases—mostly heart disease, but also diabetes, many cancers, and age-related conditions such as vision impairment, memory loss, and arthritis.

This connection between improved health and weight loss is at the core of the diet. One reason for the link is obvious. It makes absolutely no sense to adopt a weight-loss diet that isn't healthy (although, sad to say, it's been done far too often).

The other reason is the key to your success. The Sonoma Diet stresses wholesome, great-tasting foods that satisfy your hunger while delivering an abundant supply of health-inducing nutrients in a minimum number of calories. By making every calorie count, the diet intertwines health and weight loss. One ensures the other.

What people are saying about Sonoma ...

"If you only think about what you're eating when confronted with a menu board in the fast-food drive-through ... it's time to take back your power to make healthier choices. With the Sonoma Diet, I can spend 20 minutes in the kitchen cooking my way back to more flavourful food, a better nutritional balance, and a healthier weight."

Bob, age 50, weight loss to date: 14 lb

True Love

You may have trouble thinking of healthy eating as something to enjoy. That's understandable. There's a long and sometimes deserved tradition of thinking of "health food" as something unappetizing, consisting of dishes of (as Woody Allen once put it) "mashed yeast."

Let's disavow you of that caricature. The Mediterraneans have shown that the healthiest of food choices make for the tastiest of dishes. Sonoma cuisine took that idea to the next level. The Sonoma Diet brings it home to you. Skip ahead if you like and thumb through the recipes you'll be eating. You'll see what we mean. (And there's no mashed yeast in any of them.)

Many also wonder how much enjoyment is left in a diet that excludes three things they think they love the most. They're talking about sugar, saturated fat, and refined flour foods such as white bread, cereals, crackers, pasta, and cake.

That's a legitimate concern. And it's true that those ingredients, which are found exclusively in highly processed foods, are to be avoided. The simple fact is that if you want to shed pounds, you have to forget about those foods until you reach your target weight. And if you want to stay at your target weight and be healthy, those foods will be rare throughout Wave 3 of the diet—which is to say for the rest of your life.

You'll soon discover that you can easily do without white bread, fatty burgers, and sugary desserts. What you took as love was really just infatuation. Because of the way processed foods such as white bread and refined sugar affect your metabolism, eating them is more a matter of habit than enjoyment.

You're going to break yourself of those habits on Wave 1 of the diet. That will liberate you to appreciate the true joy of fresh, healthy food. Trust us, the crunch of a cool fresh apple is a far richer delight than the crunch of the twentieth potato crisp. The taste and feel of a steamy cod fillet melting in your mouth is much more sensuous than anything artery-clogging butter can offer. The chewy taste experience of whole grain bread or cereal goes way beyond the compulsive, rote experience of gobbling down white crackers or sugar-laden cereal.

And once you've learned to truly savour the natural sweetness of fresh ripe berries, then cakes, pies, and cookies will seem way too sugary.

Healthy pleasures last longer than guilty pleasures. You'll see.

WHOLE GRAINS

You've already been introduced to whole grains as a top power food in the Sonoma Diet. They qualify for the honour because of their rich fibre content and abundance of healthy nutrients, including antioxidants, vitamin E, selenium, magnesium, and B vitamins.

There's another major reason whole grains are so essential for weight loss. By eating whole grains instead of

EATING: The Sonoma Diet Way

Much of the new territory shouldn't be all that unfamiliar, either. Bran flakes instead of corn flakes, whole grain bread instead of spongy white bread, brown rice instead of white rice, porridge instead of pancakes. Most of us have been there and done that at least a few times in our lives.

refined white flour, you are sharply reducing the top metabolic cause of weight gain. The process of milling grains into white flour (or white rice, white pasta, etc.) not only robs them of most of their nutrients, it also modifies an otherwise healthy food into a quick supplier of body fat.

Here's why: all carbohydrates—grains, fruits, vegetables, and other foods—supply energy by bringing sugars into the bloodstream. Your body releases the hormone insulin to process those sugars into usable energy. What can't be used in due time is stored as body fat.

That's all fine and natural. But refined foods such as table sugar and white bread are digested and absorbed much more quickly, with damaging consequences. For starters, over time this increases the risk for heart disease and diabetes. It also makes it easier for the body to convert extra calories to body fat. The other negative factor is that what was minutes before an excess of blood sugar is now a low blood sugar level. You're soon craving more of the same refined sugar and flour that caused the problem in the first place.

Refined grains, then, are the opposite of a power food. They deliver very few nutrients at a high cost of calories that quickly become body fat.

Finding and Buying Whole Grains

On the Sonoma Diet, you eat only whole grains and never milled or refined grains. Whole grain means every part of the grain is still there. Refined grain means some has been removed, usually the fibre-rich bran (outer layer), the energy-containing endosperm (middle layer), and/or the nutrient-packed germ (inner layer).

We live in a refined grain world, so it's not always easy to know if you are in fact getting real whole grain bread or cereal. Here's what to know when you're shopping:

• Healthy-sounding words like "100% wheat," "multigrain," or "cracked wheat" have nothing to do with whether the bread or cereal is whole grain or not.

• Look for 100% whole grain or whole wheat on the ingredient label.

• Check the ingredients label. The first grain listed should be identified as "whole," and there should be no grain listed not identified as "whole."

• Don't be fooled by dark brown colouring. That can come from molasses or food colour.

• The best type of whole wheat bread advertises the term "whole cracked wheat." But remember that wheat is not the only healthy whole grain for bread or cereal.

• Choose whole grain breads with at least 2 grams of fibre per slice and whole grain cereals with at least 8 grams of fibre per serving. You'll find the fibre count in the ingredients box on the label.

Substituting whole grains for refined grains subtracts a problem food from your diet and adds a healthy, satisfying food that's conducive to weight loss.

Whole Grains for Your Health

If you're typical, white bread and crackers are old dietary friends. So switching from refined white flour products to natural whole grains may be a major change. But like any change for the better, the challenge comes only at the beginning. You'll soon see whole grains are richer tasting, offer much more variety, have a chewy, substantial feel in your mouth, and help you feel full and satisfied sooner and for longer.

Whole grains offer health benefits as well. Because whole grains keep blood sugar and insulin under control, you not only avoid needless weight gain, you also reduce your risk of diabetes, cancer, stroke, and heart disease. The evidence for this is consistent and convincing.

For example, the Harvard School of Public Health conducted a six-year study of 65,000 women and found those whose diets were high in white bread, white rice, and pasta had two and a half times the risk for type 2 ("adult onset") diabetes than those who ate a diet rich in high-fibre foods such as whole wheat breads and other whole grain items. Those who ate mostly whole grains (the daily equivalent of a bowl of porridge and two slices of whole grain bread) were 30% less likely to develop type 2 diabetes.

Whole grains also protect against heart disease, which happens to be the number one killer of American women today. Another team of Harvard researchers studied 75,000 women and concluded that those who ate more whole grains (two and a half servings per day) were 30% less likely to develop heart disease than women who ate the least.

The third major study, the Harvard

COOKING: The Sonoma Diet Way

Try a variety of cooking methods. For example, grains can be toasted in the oven for crispy treats, simmered or boiled (porridge-style), or stir-fried into "grain medleys" for salads, as a side dish, or even in a starring role as the main course. See page 287–289 for grain medley recipes.

SHOPPING: The Sonoma Diet Way

When selecting bread, read the label and make sure not only that the bread is 100% whole grain, but also that it contains at least 2 grams of fibre per slice. Otherwise, it's not a dense enough power food.

Nurses' Health Study, found that women who ate more whole grains weighed less than women who consumed fewer. Interestingly, in this study weight gain was associated with eating more refined grains.

Great Grains

Most of us hear the word "grains" and think of bread and cereal first, then maybe crackers and pasta. That's fine. The whole grain versions of those foods can be regulars in your meals. Just make sure they are indeed whole grain and not refined and that you don't exceed the serving sizes recommended in the next chapter.

But think about variety as well. Variety is not only the spice of life—it's the spirit of the Sonoma Diet. We'll be offering some alternative ways to prepare your grain allotment for each meal. You'll also want to try new and different whole grains, taking full advantage of the booming variety now available in markets. Even whole wheat, which is the most familiar whole grain, comes in different forms—such as wheat berries, bulgur, groats, and cracked wheat.

Those same variations are found in whole wheat breads as well. In fact, with a little poking around, you can eat whole wheat bread for months and never have the same kind twice. And, of course, there are other whole grain breads besides wheat, such as oat, rye, and pumpernickel. As long as it's whole grain and not refined at all, any one is fine.

Similarly, there are now many varieties of whole grain rice available, such as Chinese black rice, red rice, and brown basmati rice. All are superb vitamin B sources, and they also contain phytonutrients in the same categories as some fruits and vegetables. Another option is wild rice, a wonderfully wholesome food you may have tried only in restaurants. Brown and wild rice take a little more effort to prepare than cover-it-and-forget-it white rice, but it's worth it—for your taste and for your waist.

Pasta has a well-deserved bad reputation in weight-loss circles, but that only applies to regular wheat

SHOPPING: The Sonoma Diet Way

An alternative to whole grain pasta is now readily available in most grocery stores. Made with multigrains and legumes, it tastes and looks more like traditional refined grain pasta but with improved nutritional value.

pasta (and, of course, to any pasta in excessive amounts). Whole wheat pasta is healthy and recommended. It's also enjoying something of a boom in popularity in recent years. Or try a whole grain or nutrient-rich pasta, similar in taste to a typical pasta but rich in protein, fibre, and other nutrients.

For a change of pace from typical pasta, try a recipe from the Sonoma Diet featuring soba noodles. These are basically buckwheat noodles or pasta, an excellent whole grain alternative to refined wheat flour noodles or pasta (buckwheat isn't actually wheat at all). It's a favourite in Japan and has caught on in North America as well in recent years.

You'll also notice on the Sonoma Diet Grains list a perhaps unfamiliar entry called quinoa (pronounced keen-wa). It's a wheat alternative from South America, with a nutty taste. Grains are primarily carbohydrate with some protein as a bonus, but quinoa offers something few grains can—the same high-quality protein you get with meat or eggs. It's usually prepared like a light, fluffy rice, but you can also toast quinoa on a sheet pan in the oven. If you haven't tasted quinoa yet, try the recipe for Toasted Quinoa Pilaf on page 175.

Finally, you have your whole grain cold cereals to enjoy with fat-free milk in the morning. There's plenty to choose from among commercial brands. Make sure, however, to check the label for high fibre content. Any cereal on the Sonoma Diet should have at least 8 grams of fibre per serving. Check the label on the box for specific amounts.

VEGETABLES

We can thank the people of the Mediterranean for bringing to the North American diet a new appreciation of vegetables—but we can also appreciate the Sonoma cuisine and their local chefs for giving us insight on how to enjoy these vegetables with contemporary flavours and preparations. These preparations are not just a treasure trove of health and longevity but are also culinary delights that are right at home on the menu of any gourmet restaurant.

Despite the best efforts of southern Europeans and the chefs of Sonoma (not to mention medical researchers), Americans in general eat too few fruits and vegetables. What they do eat, they eat in insufficient variety.

This has a lot to do with why so many people are overweight and undernourished.

Sadly, low-carb diets contribute to the problem by severely restricting fruits and vegetables, sometimes to the point of near elimination. The Sonoma Diet, on the other hand, puts vegetables at centre stage. Like the Mediterranean diet, it is plant-based. That doesn't mean it's vegetarian—you'll have plenty of meat and fish—but it does mean that many of your calories will come from nutrient-rich foods such as vegetables, grains, fruits, nuts, and plant oils. Remember that all of the Sonoma Diet Top Ten Power Foods from the last chapter were from plant sources.

And seven of those 10 are fruits or vegetables. You'll lose weight because we'll show you how to take advantage of these and other nutrient-rich power foods to supply your body with all the health-promoting nutrients it needs with a calorie count small enough to let you lose weight.

The secret to getting the full health and weight-loss benefits of vegetables is to enjoy eating them. The days of considering vegetables a necessary evil on your plate are over. The recipes you'll be following stress the innate flavours of whole vegetables and the herbs and spices that go with them. You'll develop a new appreciation for the natural goodness of fresh vegetables.

Most dieters are vaguely aware that vegetables are "good for you." But eating more fruits and vegetables will also help you lose weight. To help you understand just how important they are in the Sonoma Diet, let's take a few pages to look at what they offer. Because you won't start eating fruits until 10 days into the diet, we'll talk mostly about vegetables here. But most of the benefits apply to fruits as well.

Working Together

We've already seen how the health benefits of all power foods (whether they're in the Top Ten or not) come from the abundance of plant nutrients—phytochemicals—they deliver to your cells. Research in recent years has been successful in identifying those phytonutrients, especially the ones that protect your cells by acting as antioxidants. So a question naturally arises: if we know what the beneficial chemicals in the foods are, why don't we just take them in capsule form?

As you probably know, such supplements exist. Quercetin, beta-carotene, and lycopene supplements are already popular. There are many others.

But they do little for your weight-loss goals. The whole idea of the Sonoma Diet is to satisfy your hunger by eating foods with a maximum of nutrients. Supplements certainly qualify as nutrient rich—lots of nutrients, not many calories—but they hardly make for enjoyable eating. No hunger was ever satisfied by swallowing a pill.

The other problem with supplements is that they isolate the most active nutrients. Or they supply various nutrients in unnatural proportions. This sabotages much of the benefit of nutrient-rich vegetables.

Why? Because nutritionists are convinced by the evidence that vitamins, minerals, and phytonutrients in any one vegetable work in harmony to strengthen your cardiovascular system, slow age-related vision loss, help prevent certain cancers, or deliver all their other health benefits. Separating out one phytonutrient, no matter how powerful it is, ruins this synergy. You have a solo player instead of the orchestra.

That's why whole, fresh vegetables are your best choice. This doesn't mean they can't be cooked, or that some parts can never be removed for a more pleasing dish. But you want to leave the entire line-up of phytonutrients intact as much as possible.

Towards that end, frozen vegetables are usually okay. But canned vegetables have often been processed at the expense of their nutrients. They may also contain added ingredients, such as salt, preservatives, or even saturated fat. If you must choose canned vegetables, check the ingredients list carefully.

What Eating Lots of Fruits and Vegetables Does for You

- Decreases your risk for stroke and heart attack.
- Helps protect against several types of cancers.
- Lowers blood pressure.
- Improves digestion and discourages intestinal disorders.
- Guards against cataracts and other age-related vision problems.
- Saves your memory as you grow older.
- Helps you lose weight by providing vital nutrients with a minimum of calories.

In Praise of Variety

Not only do phytochemicals work synergistically within the same vegetable, their health benefits accumulate with each kind of vegetable you eat. That's the biggest argument for the variety we advocate so strongly on the Sonoma Diet. The wider variety of vegetables you eat, the bigger the roster of plant nutrients you benefit from.

Another reason for eating lots of different vegetables, of course, is the new taste adventure each one offers. Eating a wide selection of vegetables and cooking them in subtly different ways makes every meal a taste adventure.

If you look at the three lists of recommended vegetables in the Sonoma Diet, you'll be able to group them by colours roughly according to the following categories.

SHOPPING: The Sonoma Diet Way

The easiest way to get variety into your vegetable selection is to choose a variety of colours. Generally speaking, vegetables in one colour group —red, yellow, green, etc.—contain distinct types of phytochemicals, though there is much overlap. Putting different-coloured vegetables on your plate, and changing colours again with the next meal, ensures the widest variety of nutrients while keeping your palate entertained. The Roasted Vegetable Medley (page 184) brings the brightest of yellow, orange, and red colours to the plate.

Green Vegetables

If you remember what spinach and broccoli offer as Top Ten Sonoma Diet Power Foods, you have a pretty good idea of the potency of the phytonutrients in green vegetables. Besides protecting against heart disease and cancer, eating green vegetables keeps your vision sharp and your bones and teeth strong as you get older.

The strongest members of the green team are the cruciferous vegetables— broccoli, Brussels sprouts, cabbage, kale, and pak choi. (Cauliflower is also a cruciferous vegetable, but it plays for the white team.) These vegetables are especially rich in a huge variety of antioxidant phytonutrients, as well as vitamins and minerals.

SHOPPING: The Sonoma Diet Way

A quick and easy way to get a variety of fresh greens is to pick up different versions of the bagged salad blends available at supermarkets.

Another sub-category consists of green, leafy vegetables that are usually used in salads but can also be sautéed, stir-fried, or steamed. Spinach is the top power food among these greens, but there are many others. Examples include kale and mustard greens and the tops of turnips and beetroots. Many of the green vegetables and dark leafy greens such as chard, kale, Brussels sprouts, rocket, and dandelion have bitter flavours that are not too

Salads That Satisfy

A tossed salad of fresh vegetables mixed with greens is an ideal food for the Sonoma Diet. It works to fulfil the vegetable requirement in any meal instruction. We'll even look the other way if you pile your salad a little too high in Wave 2.

Be sure to power pack your salads with nutrient-rich raw vegetables. Experiment with different ingredients to wake up that salad and turn it into a tasty treat.

• Iceberg is an old standby, but it's the least nutrient-rich lettuce there is. Essentially it's just an empty vehicle for salad dressing. Try something else.

• The darker the green you use, the more nutrient-rich it usually is. Romaine and watercress, for example, have eight times more beta-carotene and twice the calcium and potassium as iceberg.

• Other good dark green leaf choices are spinach, beetroot greens, turnip greens, kale, and mustard greens.

• Try the unfamiliar. A number of European or Asian greens are now available in UK markets. Rocket, sorrel, chicory (also called endive), frisée, mizuna, and tatsoi are delicious, nutritious, and a worthwhile change of pace.

• There's no rule saying that salad greens have to be green. Try radicchio (wine red) and Belgian endive (purple).

• Add those raw Top Ten Sonoma Diet Power Foods into your salads—peppers of all colours, almonds, broccoli (or broccoli sprouts), tomatoes, spinach, even sliced grapes or toasted grains.

• Olive oil- and/or vinaigrette-based dressings are a big part of the Sonoma Diet. Remember that extra-virgin olive oil improves the flavours of all greens and helps your body absorb their nutrients. Or try using nut oils and flavour-infused vinegars to add some variety to your salad dressings.

popular, to say the least. These bitter flavours happen to be the personality of their powerful antioxidants. When they are prepared in the right company of ingredients, the bitterness mellows to a delicious flavour and your body can absorb these antioxidants better. Try preparing these vegetables with ingredients such as olive oil, nuts, lemon juice, or small amounts of flavourful cheeses. Look through the Sonoma Diet recipes for more ideas.

> **EATING: The Sonoma Diet Way**
> You can use radicchio to add colour and a distinct taste to your salads. You can also stir-fry it in a little olive oil or even grill it.

Red Vegetables

Radishes, red peppers, red onions, and beetroots head up this category. Red vegetables are especially helpful in preserving memory function and urinary tract health, as well as protecting against heart disease and cancer.

Tomatoes, with their lycopene content, are the most powerful red vegetables. Keep in mind that to get the most benefit from tomatoes' phytonutrients, it's better to cook them (skin and all) and accompany the stew or sauce with olive oil. That helps your body's absorption of the lycopene and also boosts the flavour and sweetness of the tomatoes themselves.

If you haven't tried radicchio, make sure you do. It's a wine red leafy vegetable from Italy that's now popular and readily available in the UK. Its star nutrient, a phytochemical called intybin, aids digestion and strengthens the liver.

White Vegetables

Cauliflower, turnips, onions, and mushrooms jump to mind when you think of white vegetables. So do some flavour enhancers such as ginger and garlic. All are excellent power foods—lots of great taste and healthy nutrients for a tiny amount of calories.

Onions are especially good heart protectors. They share with garlic a powerful phytonutrient called allicin, which helps prevent atherosclerosis, or hardening of the arteries.

Jicama (HEE-ka-mah) is a fleshy white root (under a brown skin) that can be steamed, baked, or boiled like a potato. It's also a light and tasty treat eaten raw. Cut it into cubes and try it as a snack with fruit or mixed with green salads. Try cutting jicama into sticks and dipping it in Hummus, a recipe from the Sonoma Diet Seasonings section on page 149.

Yellow and Orange Vegetables

These are especially effective in protecting your vision and immune system. Carrots, sweetcorn, swede, several squashes, and the yellow or orange versions of tomatoes and peppers are members of this colour family.

Here you'll find some of the most beneficial phytonutrient categories, such as the antioxidant carotenoids and flavonoids. These are also examples of vegetables that contain antioxidants, which will perform better for you when combined with healthy types of fats. Interestingly, some of the yellow and orange vegetables are relatively high in natural sugars, which is why they are Tier 2 or 3 vegetables.

Purple Vegetables

Yes, there are purple vegetables. Had you forgotten aubergine, Belgian endive, and red cabbage? You'll also find purple-colour peppers, purple asparagus, and even purple carrots. The phytonutrients responsible for the colour (usually in the phenol or anthocyanin category) seem to be helpful in slowing down the ravages of ageing. Urinary tract health and memory function benefit from purple vegetables. If you're looking for a tasty way to fix aubergine, the Roasted Aubergine Salad on page 178 is a good start.

FATS

Dietary fat is what you eat. Body fat is what you want to reduce. Dietary fat can lead to body fat, but not as directly or inevitably as you may have assumed.

The Sonoma Diet fat philosophy is simple. The right kind of dietary fat in the right amounts is not only good for your health but vital to your weight loss. Very low-fat diets will not work for most people. Researchers from Harvard found that people following a Mediterranean-style diet for weight loss were more successful than those following a low-fat diet. The types of fats eaten in this diet were primarily monounsaturated: peanut butter, nuts, and olive and canola oils. What is the message here? The tastier and more satisfying the food, the greater the overall success. Another interesting find in this study was that the quality of the diet within the Mediterranean groups was far better and more nutrient rich than the low-fat diet. You need to maintain the right balance between fats, proteins, and carbohydrates in order to shed pounds in a healthy way. The meal plans you'll be following on the Sonoma Diet are designed to do just that.

The reasons you need fats in your diet are many—mainly for health, flavour, and enjoyment. We've already seen how extra-virgin olive oil and nuts, the star fats from the Mediterranean diet, actually lower levels of the bad LDL cholesterol and deliver heart-healthy nutrients. Other fats, such as avocados, peanuts, and omega-3 oils (found in salmon, walnuts, and flaxseeds), also provide beneficial nutrients such as antioxidants and phytonutrients.

Just as important, fats help you feel just full enough as you finish a meal. Without that feeling of satiety, you'll eventually start overeating just to find some kind of satisfaction. Anyone who's been on a very low-fat diet knows that feeling well.

Fats also increase the benefits of other nutrient-rich foods. For example,

---

The Ugly Fat

If extra-virgin olive oil is the good and saturated fat is the bad, then partially hydrogenated fat is the ugly. This altered fat is found in processed food, fried food, margarine, and many kinds of packaged baked foods such as cakes, biscuits, tarts, and pies.

Also called trans fats, partially hydrogenated fats are chemically altered oils that are solid and creamy. Originally conceived as an inexpensive alternative to saturated fats, partially hydrogenated fats are even more damaging to your heart and overall health.

Avoid them at all costs. Buy fresh foods instead of packaged items and you'll never run across this type of fat. If you do buy packaged or processed foods, check the label. If the words "partially hydrogenated" fat or oil, "trans fat," or "trans fatty acid" appear on the ingredients list or label, put the package back and buy something else.

---

lycopene, the super nutrient in tomatoes, can't be properly absorbed in your digestive tract without some dietary fat in the vicinity. A strategic, nutrient-boosting use of fats is one of the secrets of the Mediterranean diet. Italians, to choose an obvious example, know full well the value of combining tomato sauce and olive oil.

And last but not least, don't underestimate the value of fats as flavour. The Sonoma Diet Fats are recommended for use to add flavour to your meals. The recipes are created with that in mind. Remember, enjoying your meals is crucial.

In fact, there's evidence that certain types of dietary fat have a mood-elevating function. Restaurant chefs are certainly aware of that. Unfortunately, the answer is not in emptying tubs of butter into cooking pans. On the other hand, chefs today, particularly in the Sonoma and neighbouring Napa Valley wine regions, are inspired by the Mediterranean diet and the health-conscious lifestyle of their own region. Their focus is on quality ingredients with a balanced use of healthy fats, herbs, and spices to create flavour and health in food. That's what you'll be doing too.

There's Fat and Then There's Fat

As the title tells us, not all fats were created alike. There are three naturally occurring types of fat: saturated, monounsaturated, and polyunsaturated, as well as one manufactured fat, known as hydrogenated oil (commonly referred to as trans fat).

The majority of the types of fat you should eat come mostly from plant oils. The healthiest are led by monounsaturated fats, such as extra-virgin olive oil, nuts, canola oil, and avocados. Other healthy oils are found in the polyunsaturated category, such as grapeseed oil, sunflower oil, and the omega-3 oils found in some cold-water fish, flaxseeds, and walnuts.

The kind of fat you must limit eating is the saturated fat found mostly in animal foods such as meats and dairy products, as well as those found in palm and coconut oils. This does not mean you can't eat meat or dairy. You can. But it does mean that you must seek the lean or non-fat versions of meat or dairy foods.

You can recognize saturated fat because it's solid at room temperature or lower—the white rimming a steak, the marble in prime rib, the chicken fat that skims a soup in the fridge, a stick of butter. Its primary sin is raising the levels of bad LDL cholesterol in your arteries, inviting heart disease. In fact, saturated fat ups your blood cholesterol more than dietary cholesterol itself. Hydrogenated oils should be avoided because they have far worse effects on your health and heart than saturated fats.

Omega-3 Benefits

Omega-3 oils have a long history of protecting the immune system and play a role in protecting the body from heart disease, depression, Alzheimer's disease, diabetes, inflammation, colitis, psoriasis, and arthritis.

Fat Balance

A closer look to the meaning of "balance" also applies to the quality and amounts of these types of dietary fats eaten. As you have already learned, the type of fat you eat is more of an issue than the actual amount of fat you eat.

The saying "you are what you eat" holds absolute truth. A closer look within your body reflects the types of fats you eat on a daily basis. These fats or fatty acids make up the outer covering of cells, known as cell membranes. Depending on the type, balance, and amount of fats eaten, immune systems can be influenced, raising or lowering the risk for inflammation, heart disease, diabetes, arthritis, cancer, and even depression.

What exactly does this balance involve? This means eating primarily from the monounsaturated fat category, consuming lesser amounts of vegetable oils such as corn oil and soya bean oil, eating saturated fats to an even lesser degree, and avoiding hydrogenated oils. In the last century, Americans have drastically increased their intake of processed foods and vegetable oils in relation to the intake of omega-3 oils. An increased consumption of vegetable seed oils makes it difficult for the body to reap the benefits of the omega-3 oils. For many who already consume low amounts of these omega-3-rich foods, this poses an even greater disadvantage. Omega-3-rich foods include salmon, mackerel, tuna, flaxseeds, soya, and walnuts.

Nuts to You

Eating nuts several times a week has been shown to help reduce your risk of heart disease by 30 to 50%. How much should you eat? About a handful of nuts, or 25 g/1 oz per serving, provides a great source of protein—almost as much as you'll find in most meats. Nuts are great as snacks and perfect taste boosters when sprinkled on salads or added to hot dishes. They're almost as calorie rich as they are nutrient rich, so you'll be eating them in measured amounts. You'll appreciate that. Small servings of nuts allow you to savour their special taste rather than gobbling them down thoughtlessly. Remember, nuts do contain a hefty number of calories, so don't overdo it. Nut portions should be determined according to your meal plan.

You've already met nutrient-rich almonds, a Top Ten Power Food on the Sonoma Diet. There are also other nuts on the Sonoma Diet Fats list—walnuts, peanuts, and pecans (although other nuts can be substituted). Each contains all three kinds of fat, including the preferred monounsaturated fats.

Walnut trees abound in Sonoma, as they do along the Mediterranean. They're almost the prototype of a healthy nut. Walnuts are the richest plant source (as opposed to fish) of omega-3 fatty acids. Besides cardiovascular protection, walnuts promote cognitive function (such as memory) and have an anti-inflammatory effect that helps fight respiratory problems, arthritis, and skin conditions.

Walnuts, almonds, peanuts, and extra-virgin olive oil are foods you'd be asked to eliminate on a low-fat diet. On the Sonoma Diet, you'll be encouraged to use them often.

Protein

There's going to be protein in one form or another on your plate at every meal, every day. If you look ahead at the Sonoma Diet Proteins and Dairy list (page 75 for Wave 1 and page 92 for Wave 2), you'll see that you have a huge number of choices for meeting that requirement. Variety is the magic word for protein as much as it is for fruits, vegetables, and grains.

Meat and Fish

Meat is a perfectly acceptable protein choice on the Sonoma Diet. It has the advantage of being a "complete" protein, meaning it provides your body with all the amino acids (protein components) it needs. Any individual plant protein source, with the exception of quinoa and soya, can't quite do that. So if you're vegetarian, you need more variety to make sure all amino acids are covered. Plus, meat provides dietary iron in a form that is most easily absorbed by your body.

Your main consideration in choosing meats is leanness. Any cut of meat that's too high in saturated fat will do you and your diet more harm than good.

The "lean" requirement rules out a number of meat choices completely. Bacon, sausage, dark poultry, brisket, offal, and rib steak are just too fat-riddled, no matter how you cut them. You won't be eating them until you reach your target weight, and even then only once in a blue moon.

That still leaves a lot of meat choices—from lamb, veal, and venison to beef, pork, and white poultry meat (always without the skin). But none of those is going to automatically be lean enough to suit your weight-loss needs. Make sure you choose the leanest cuts.

Fish, of course, is another meat alternative. It's a lower-calorie alternative to other meats, with all the protein, nutrients, and in some cases omega-3 oils. Don't forget shellfish for even more variety.

SHOPPING: The Sonoma Diet Way

One way to be smart about meat consumption is to limit yourself to the specific lean cuts of beef (or pork, lamb, or veal) designated on the Sonoma Diet Proteins and Dairy list (page 75 for Wave 1; page 92 for Wave 2). These have been carefully selected as lean cuts. A very lean cut of beef can have four times less saturated fat than a fatty cut and deliver more protein at half the calories. That's how you lose weight.

Eggs

Another fine protein choice is eggs. They don't deliver quite as much protein per calorie as most meat cuts, but more of their fat is monounsaturated. What's more, the yolks turn out to be a good source of easily absorbable lutein, the eye-saving carotenoid found in spinach and other green vegetables.

By the way, eggs' undeserved reputation for increasing cholesterol levels in the bloodstream has been thoroughly debunked. One recent study found no difference in heart disease risk between those who ate one egg a week and those who ate one a day. Another concluded that eating two eggs a day for six weeks had no impact at all on cholesterol levels. However, what is important is how you prepare your eggs. Large amounts of butter, cheese, and cream in the company of sausage and bacon don't lead to weight loss.

Other Protein Choices

Animal foods aren't your only protein choices. Soya beans are the top plant food for protein. They're also rich in genistein, a type of plant nutrient in the isoflavone phytonutrient category. It acts much like a plant-based oestrogen and is thought to be protective against breast cancer in women and prostate cancer in men.

Soya also has the advantage of changing shapes and forms to suit any taste. Besides the beans themselves or tofu, there are any number of soya substitutes. Natural food manufacturers have been able to use soya to mimic the texture and taste of an amazing selection of meat products, including burgers, bacon, and crumbles. Edamame, which are fresh soya beans, are wonderful as a snack, salad, or with a grain medley.

You can also use certain legumes and beans as proteins. They include chickpeas, lentils, and lima, black, kidney, and pinto beans. These foods are mostly carbohydrates, so their protein-to-calorie ratio is not ideal. But they're a reasonable Wave 2 protein choice for vegetarians.

Dairy foods such as cheese and milk pack plenty of protein. However, they are listed separately from the other protein foods and cannot be used to fill a protein requirement in your meal instructions. Use dairy only when the meal instructions call for dairy.

Dairy is a minor player in the Sonoma Diet. Because it's so often full of saturated fat, your portions are limited. You can put fat-free milk on your whole grain cereal in the mornings or occasionally choose lower-fat cheeses such as Parmesan, mozzarella, feta, goat's cheese, and cottage cheese. You can also find low-fat cheeses, such as Cheddar. In addition, you can occasionally use small amounts of strongly flavoured cheeses such as blue cheese to add richness and flavour to meals. These strong-flavoured cheeses can go a long way in small amounts.

WAVE 1

You probably have a pretty good idea by now of the special qualities that make this diet work. You've learned the approach that distinguishes the Sonoma Diet from others. You've met the food. You know the emphasis on the vastly improved health that goes hand in hand with weight loss.

Now it's time to get started. Ready to shed some pounds?

You'll begin with Wave 1, the first of three diet segments. Each wave is designed slightly differently based on what works best for you and your body at each stage of your progress.

Wave 1 is only for 10 days. Its main goal is to introduce you to the pleasures of fine, but simple, meals. You will immediately start eating delicious breakfasts, lunches, and dinners prepared with healthy whole foods.

Your whole attitude about food will change. A meal will no longer be something to be consumed quickly without much thought. Your food will instead be appreciated as a treasured gift from nature to be savoured slowly.

At the same time, Wave 1 will rid you of three destructive eating habits that cause weight gain. The first is an overdependence on highly refined foods that turn your metabolism into a body fat production factory. Sugary desserts, white bread and crackers, sweetened cereals, and the like will be replaced by healthier but equally satisfying alternatives, mainly whole grains.

The second habit you'll lose is the haphazard eating of whatever happens to be available, easy, or familiar. This may be comfortable in the short run, but it's unsatisfying in the long run and keeps you overweight. Balanced meals with the right combination of food types are a prerequisite for healthy weight loss. Balanced meals are just as easy to make as the old grab-and-eat method because we've done the balancing for you. Your only job is to follow the simple meal plans or use the plate diagrams and food lists we give you.

The third bad habit you'll lose is (to put it bluntly) eating too much. Overeating isn't something most people do intentionally. A lot of overweight people have no idea they're overdoing it with the portions. It all seems so normal.

But if you have pounds to lose, chances are pretty good your portions have crept up toward the generous side over the years. Wave 1 will set your meal sizes at where they need to be to leave you satisfied but still on the road to weight loss. Portion control might be a bit of a challenge at first, but you can do it. In fact, one of the most common reactions from new dieters on the Sonoma Diet is genuine surprise at how filling and satisfying the adjusted portion sizes are after a few days.

To get you on the right track, we'll give you explicit and precise instructions about how much of each food type to eat with each meal. We'll even tell you exactly how much room each food type will take up on your plate. You can't go wrong.

The 10 days of Wave 1 bring your most rapid weight loss. You will at first be very aware of the adjusted portion size and the absence of long-familiar habit foods. But you will also discover the pleasure of quality food and Sonoma-style recipes. And you'll be inspired by the quick weight loss. You'll feel your life changing for the better.

GETTING SONOMA DIET-READY

The first day you start following the Wave 1 meal plans in this chapter will be considered Day 1 of your diet. There will be 10 such days in Wave 1. But even before Day 1 comes Day 0. This is the fun day.

Day 0 is the day you turn your life around—away from the unhealthy and disheartening old habits of weight gain and towards a new lifestyle of pleasurable, healthy eating for weight loss. You'll do this with a symbolic gesture that also serves as practical preparation for your new way of eating. It requires a rubbish bin, recycling bins, several boxes, and about a week's worth of grocery money.

Bring the bins right into your kitchen. They should be empty (though they won't be for long). Set the boxes down on the kitchen table or pantry. You'll be filling them with gifts for your neighbours or donations to the local homeless centre.

Make sure the kids are out of the house. They won't want to see this.

Out with the Old . . .

Now start going through the food in your pantries and shelves. Packaged goods are the least likely to survive the purge, so start with them. Check the ingredients list. If it includes refined wheat or any other processed grains, put it in the gift box or throw it away. If there's hydrogenated fat in it, get rid of it. If there's added sugar, it's out of there.

You've probably just expelled every bread, cake, biscuit, cracker, and packaged sweet from your kitchen. Good. That's what you want.

All those long bags of spaghetti and other pastas made from refined wheat? Gone. The instant macaroni and cheese packages? Gone. The bags of white rice that have been accumulating because you kept buying new ones when there was still plenty left in the old ones? Gone. The sugar-coated flakes, the fruity puffs—and any other non-whole grain cereal, whether it's sugary or not? Gone.

Bags of sugar must go for sure. Hide the honey—you can't have it around until you move to Wave 2. Potato crisps? Corn chips? Bye-bye. Tortillas? Adios.

Your spice cabinet contents are safe. So is your coffee and tea bag supply.

Now turn your attention to the bottles. Look especially for saturated or hydrogenated fats on the ingredients labels. Toss the mayonnaise, unless it's made with canola oil. Mustard can stay, as can any type of vinegar. But any creamy salad dressings have to go. So do any oils that aren't extra-virgin olive oil or nut oils. Toss high-sugar bottled marinades.

Kitchen Clean-up

These foods will have to go:

- Sugar
- Bread (except Whole Grain)
- Cake and Cake Mix
- Biscuits
- Crackers (except Whole Grain)
- Packaged desserts
- White Rice
- Cereal (except Whole Grain)
- Crisps
- Mayonnaise
- Creamy Salad Dressings
- Oils (except Extra-Virgin Olive Oil and Nut Oils)
- Lard
- Regular Fizzy Drinks
- Fruit Juices
- Jam and Jelly
- Maple Syrup
- Margarine
- Butter
- Full-fat Cheese and Cream Cheese
- Ice Cream
- Milk (except Fat-free)
- Fatty Meats such as Bacon or Sausages
- Fruit (unless it can be frozen for later use)

Check food labels for the following ingredients and remove them from your kitchen:

- Refined Wheat
- Processed Grains
- Hydrogenated Fat
- Saturated Fat
- Sugar
- Refined Flour

The wine you'll keep, but put it away for 10 days. Also store your liquor collection. You won't be touching it until you reach your target weight.

Fizzy drinks, fruit juices, fruit drinks, jams, jellies, maple syrup, molasses, marshmallows, sweets—they all belong to the neighbours now. Their kids will love you.

Right about now, you're probably thinking that this kitchen cleansing is kind of fun. There is indeed something cathartic about literally throwing out your bad habits. And you haven't even got to the refrigerator yet!

In the fridge, the rules are the same. Anything with refined flour, saturated or hydrogenated fat, or sugar needs to be tossed out. That means margarine, butter, cream cheese, cream, lard, yogurt, and ice cream. Any milk that's not fat-free has to go. The eggs can stay. So can any meat that's on the Sonoma Diet Proteins and Dairy list. Fatty meats, non-Sonoma

Diet meats such as bacon, sausages, and the like must go, however.

The vegetables and fruits require a little thinking. You won't be eating fruits for 10 days, so any fresh fruits that won't last that long will have to be given away. Fruits that can be frozen—such as bananas and berries—can be spared. And of course the fruits you bought frozen in bags are safe.

As for vegetables, you'll need to check the Sonoma Diet lists. Tier 1 vegetables will stay, of course. You'll be eating them right away. But if they're on the Tier 2 or Tier 3 lists, you won't be eating any of them for 10 days. That's a long time to expect a vegetable to last. So your neighbours are probably in luck again.

Now for the final inspection. Go through what's left and make sure each surviving food item appears somewhere on the lists of acceptable Sonoma Diet Wave 1 foods—that is, any of the lists except for Tier 2 and 3 fruits and vegetables, and the sweets. If not . . . well, you know what to do. Toss 'em.

By now a thought may have occurred to you. Wouldn't it be more fun to eliminate all these forbidden foods by eating them as a grand farewell feast? Wouldn't that be less wasteful than throwing or giving them away? Well, maybe. But it sure wouldn't be in the spirit of the Sonoma Diet lifestyle.

Remember, you're not just getting rid of foods that make you fat. You're making a statement about your new way of living and eating. The thud of a sugar bag hitting the bottom of the rubbish bin makes that statement louder than an ill-advised and unhealthy food binge. Don't you think?

. . . In with the New

You're left with a kitchen with hardly any food in it. So let's fill it up. But with what?

The best guides are the lists of allowable foods (page 75), such as the Sonoma Diet Grains, the Sonoma Diet Proteins and Dairy, the Sonoma Diet Fats, and so on. Whatever is on those lists you can stock up on.

But remember that you'll be following Wave

What people are saying about Sonoma ...

"My weight loss has just started with 11 lb, but I'll take it! I like being able to look in my cupboards and fridge knowing that I can eat anything that I have in them. Having your kitchen 'Sonoma ready' takes away temptation and saves time when preparing meals. I'm surprised that the grain choices are my favourite because they are new to my eating habits, and, although it may sound a little boring, I eat vegetables at every meal."
Jean, age 57, weight loss to date: 11 lb

1 meal plans for the next 10 days, so there are some extra limits. For example, don't buy any fruits yet. No desserts yet either, even if they're unsugared. Only buy vegetables on the Tier 1 list; the other Tiers have to wait until Wave 2.

Buy only about five days' worth of vegetables. Then resupply for the final five days of Wave 1. The reason for that is the nutrients are most potent when you buy vegetables ripe and eat them soon. And don't forget variety! Remember the colour categories we went through in the last chapter? Now's your chance to do some colourful shopping.

Restocking the proteins is a trickier part of your first supply run—simply because there are so many to choose from. Where to start? Well, you'll probably want a dozen eggs. For the rest, let variety be your guide and buy enough for two or three modest protein portions per day. Because you can freeze the meat, you'll have what you need for the entire 10 days—maybe

---

Take It Easy—At Least Once a Day

The secret to weight loss is not just what you eat and how much, but in what manner. There's good evidence that more weight is gained by eating on the run or standing in front of a refrigerator than by sitting down to enjoy a sumptuous full meal.

There's even better evidence that people who eat fast are prone to overeat, since they're still bolting down the food while the stomach is sending a message to the brain that it's had enough. Fast eating also causes the same glucose-control problems with your metabolism that are such a major cause of excess body fat.

Stress-free, pleasurable eating is at the heart of the Sonoma Diet. You want to savour your meal, taste, and appreciate each bite of the delicious foods you're eating. You can't do that in a hurry. You need to slow down and make your meals a leisurely part of your life.

We know that's not always easy to do in today's fast-paced world. Your goal is to do it anyway. During Wave 1, start off by vowing to make at least one meal a day a Sonoma Diet-style meal—slow, stress-free, and pleasure-oriented. No rushing to eat, no eating on the run or standing up, no eating while talking on the phone or watching television.

One slow meal a day should be possible. Try it. Plan for it. Make the time for it. Slow eating is something you can get used to and love. It will help your weight-loss efforts.

---

some lamb, some lean beef, some fish, and poultry. Stock up on beans, lentils, and soya beans as well. You'll appreciate those when you you're not in the mood for meat, fish, or eggs.

A logical way to plan your protein purchases—and all the other foods, for that matter—is to follow the suggested meal guide for the 10 days of Wave 1. After the meal guide, you'll find the recipes you'll need and you can use these to help plan your shopping list.

Of course you may not be planning on following the meal guide to the T. You don't need to as long as you stick to the given proportions of food types. But it still makes for a handy guide for estimating what you'll need to have on hand for the next 10 days.

For your fat sources, you'll need a bottle of extra-virgin olive oil. There are tons of brands on the market; olive oil is up there with wine in its regional varieties and subtle taste differences. Buy smaller bottles so you'll have a chance to taste several alternatives over the next several weeks. You also have avocados as an option.

Also stock up on all four nuts that are approved as fat sources—almonds, walnuts, pecans, and peanuts. Buy them whole and untreated. Shelled is okay if you prefer, but not salted, fried, or mixed with other things. As with most foods in the Sonoma Diet, you want them in their natural state.

Your dairy shopping is limited. Buy some mozzarella and Parmesan. Concentrate on finding flavourful cheeses for which you won't need a lot to enjoy the full taste. Cottage cheese is good too, but choose 1% fat. You can use fat-free skimmed milk for your whole grain cereal in the morning. Fat-free plain yogurt as an alternative to skimmed milk has to wait until Wave 2. Because dairy is limited in this wave, consider taking a calcium supplement.

You'll need your grains, of course. They're part of your diet from the beginning. Refer to the tips on page 45 for buying real whole grain bread and whole grain cereals. And make sure any bread has at least 2 grams of fibre per slice and any cereal has at least 8 grams per serving. For ideas on grains to buy that are neither bread nor cereal, check the Wave 1 recipes beginning on page 166.

BREAKFAST

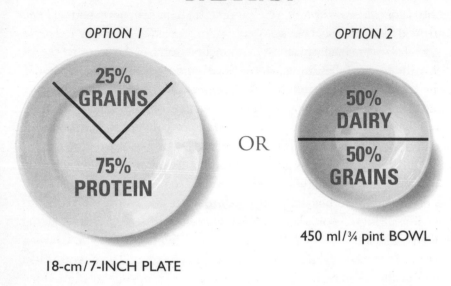

OPTION 1

25%
GRAINS

75%
PROTEIN

18-cm/7-INCH PLATE

OR

OPTION 2

50%
DAIRY

50%
GRAINS

450 ml/¾ pint BOWL

LUNCH

DINNER

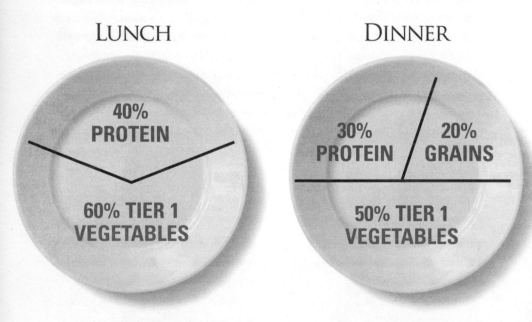

40%
PROTEIN

60% TIER 1
VEGETABLES

23-cm/9-INCH PLATE

30%
PROTEIN

20%
GRAINS

50% TIER 1
VEGETABLES

23-cm/9-INCH PLATE

A Plate (and Bowl) of Your Own

After you've filled your kitchen with a generous supply of the Sonoma Diet foods, you'll need to check the size of your family's plates and bowls. You need to know how much of the plate to cover and how much of the bowl to fill.

No need to purchase new plates and bowls. Use the same plates and bowls as the rest of your family; just measure the sizes and keep those dimensions in mind throughout your stay on the Sonoma Diet—that is, through Waves 1 and 2. Once you get to Wave 3, you'll know portion sizes so well, you'll be able to make any size plate work.

For breakfast, you'll need to pay attention to a circle 18 cm/7 inches in diameter. Your breakfast bowl (for cereals with milk or whatever else won't stay on a plate) must hold 450 ml/¾ pint of liquid—if it holds more, know where the fill line is. For lunch and dinner, you'll use a circle 23 cm/9 inches in diameter.

Remember, that's diameter—not radius or circumference. Take a ruler, bisect the plate with it, and see what it measures from edge to edge. If it's 18 cm/7 inches or 23 cm/9 inches, you have one of your plates. If it's larger, note where the 18- and 23-cm or 7- and 9-inch marks are and only use that much of the plate. For the bowl, just pour 450 ml/¾ pint of water into it. If that fills it, you've got your bowl. If more will fit in the bowl, pay attention to how much of the bowl the amount fills. Keep in mind that plate styles differ—many have an extra-wide rim that adds a bit to the diameter size of the plate. If the centre of the plate happens to be the measurement you want, just ignore the rim when you place food on the plate.

You probably already have plates and a bowl of those sizes in your collection somewhere. If so, fine. If not and you're afraid you'll overload your plate, cut a paper plate to the correct size. Place it over your regular plate before each meal to help you remember how much of your plate to use and how much to leave empty.

The reason for these picky plate-size requirements is portion control. You'll be eating the right amount of food at each meal because only the right amount will fit on your plate. The recipes and food choices are carefully designed to your plate size. So to eat right, you don't count calories or grams or anything else. You just fill your plate or bowl with the foods we recommend in the meal plans.

THE WAY OF WAVE 1

To repeat, the purpose of Wave 1 is to naturally recalibrate the body, to get you going with your new healthy eating habits, to expose you to the pleasures of delicious whole-food recipes, and to reintroduce you to reasonable portion sizes.

That's a tall order, but it's all going to happen within 10 days. That's how fast the transition is. It won't be gradual. You're going to leave behind your old habits and start losing weight on Day 1.

For that to happen, Wave 1 has to be more restrictive than Wave 2. Your portion sizes will be the same, but they'll contain fewer calories than Wave 2 portions. This is by far the most effective way to cure you of your overeating habit. Baby steps simply don't work.

The most important transition, though, will be to get you off the refined flour/white bread/sugar caravan that has wreaked so much havoc with your metabolism. You have a habit to break. You have to get those bread-and-cake cravings out of your system. The only way to do it is cold turkey.

Not that it will be a miserable experience by any means. Unlike "low-carb" and other diets, you'll still be eating bread and cereal even during Wave 1. But the slower-absorbing whole grain versions will help wean you off the white bread habit.

You will stop eating refined sugar immediately. Again, the sugar habit has to be totally eliminated or you'll continue to crave sweets and you won't lose weight. Most artificial-sugar desserts are forbidden in Wave 1, even though they don't have the same effect on your metabolism. There's a good reason for this. You won't lose your cravings if you continue to satisfy them, even with sugarless, artificially sweetened substitutes. Scientific studies suggest that even diet drinks or artificially sweetened drinks stimulate the appetite. So it's best to avoid sugar (real or artificial) completely in the first 10 days.

What people are saying about Sonoma ...

"I really like this diet. I like the fact that you are able to see results in the first week. I also like the fact that you are eating food that fills you up. I never walk away hungry, and I still have plenty of energy. That first week is the hardest, but after my body adjusted itself, the new lifestyle was not that bad. Another thing I like about this diet is that I feel I'm not losing muscles as I'm losing weight. I see that I'm getting more defined and still keeping muscle. I'm just losing the fat, which is what I want. Personally, I don't want to be skinny. I want to look healthy, and this diet helps do that."

Bruce, age 29, weight loss to date: 25 lb

But if you absolutely can't give up your diet drink, limit it to two cans per day. Same goes for sweeteners—limit to two packets per day.

Even fruits are taboo on Wave 1. Again, the reason is sugar content. The natural fruits' sugars (fructose) are generally benign because the fruits' natural fibres slow down their absorption in your digestive system. But the most important goal of Wave 1 is to break your sugar addiction, so anything that even reminds you of sweetness— even healthy fruits—needs to be put aside for the time being.

It will all be worth it. You'll be pleasantly surprised at how quickly you lose your cravings for white bread and sugary sweets. The effort you put into Wave 1 will pay off throughout Waves 2 and 3 and for the rest of your life.

You'll notice a few other Wave 1 restrictions that don't exist in Wave 2. One is wine. We encourage a glass of wine with one meal for those who enjoy it, for reasons we'll explain in the next chapter. But not during Wave 1. There are two reasons for the delay. One is that wine, made from grapes, has its own form of sugar. The other is that the lower calorie count factored into Wave 1 meals for a quick start to your weight loss simply doesn't leave room for wine. So hold off for 10 days. The pleasure will be there soon.

EATING: The Sonoma Diet Way

Cutting back all of the sugar you've been consuming since childhood isn't easy to do. Just remember: the more you give in to your cravings, the less likely you are to overcome them. Yet we also know how hard it is to quit your sugar consumption cold turkey. If you can make it through Wave 1 without consuming any sweet foods whatsoever, we hope you'll be able to continue avoiding refined sugars. Just can't take it any more? Then limit yourself to no more than 1 to 2 cans of diet drink and 1 to 2 packets of artficial sweetener per day. Don't exceed this. You'll thank yourself in the long run.

Your vegetable choices are also more limited in Wave 1. Only Tier 1 vegetables are allowed. That's because the vegetables in the higher tiers have less fibre and more natural sugars than their Tier 1 counterparts. That's not a terrible trait by any means, but it doesn't help your system get off the metabolic merry-go-round that's the top priority in Wave 1.

And one vegetable is out for the length of the diet. White potatoes have their charms and benefits, but their starchy nature makes them behave just

What to Drink

The Sonoma Diet is not big on a variety of mealtime beverages (though we do recommend drinking eight 225 ml/8 fl oz glasses of water per day). A feeling of satisfaction from eating is of primary importance, and liquids don't provide that. On Wave 1, you can drink water, teas such as green tea (the most heart-healthy of all the teas), black tea, and herbal tea (chamomile, hibiscus), as well as coffee. You'll drink a glass of wine if you wish with one meal per day when you reach Wave 2. Sugar-free fizzy drinks are also allowed—but limit yourself to two cans per day.

Why not fruit juices? Because they deliver the natural sugars of fruits without the fibre and without the full dose of nutrients. Drinking fruit juice doesn't address your psychological need to chew the way eating whole fruits does. When you drink fruit juices, you're ingesting calories without the "mouth" satisfaction that comes from chewing and swallowing. Studies consistently show that those calories from drinking juice end up added on to your overall daily calorie intake.

like white bread. You're going to have to forget about potatoes until you weigh what you want to weigh, and even then you'll want to limit how often you eat them.

How to Fill Your Plate

The actual food instructions for the Sonoma Diet are so simple that we can run through them in no time. Simply look at the plate diagrams on page 68 and fill your plate or bowl accordingly.

In Wave 1, you have three breakfast options. The first is to fill your 18-cm/7-inch plate (remember, the 23-cm/9-inch plate is only for lunch and dinner) with 75% protein and 25% whole grain. What might fit nicely, for example, is a two-egg omelette with a little diced ham for the 75% protein space and a piece of whole grain toast (no butter) for the 25% whole grain area. You can also have 100% protein—a mushroom omelette, for example. The third Wave 1 breakfast option allows you to fill your bowl with half dairy and half whole grains. The most obvious way to do that is to have some whole grain cereal with fat-free milk. It's that simple.

As long as you don't pile the food high on your plate, or go back for seconds, you've eaten according to Wave 1 recommendations.

For lunch and dinner, the choices are more substantial. You can see in the diagrams that there are two ways to fill your 23-cm/9-inch plate. One is for lunch and the other is for dinner. It doesn't matter which is which, but it should never be two of the same (because that would throw the overall proportions out of balance).

Let's say you pick for lunch the combination calling for 40% protein and 60% vegetables (only Tier 1 vegetables, because you're in Wave 1). You might want to split your 60% vegetable space between a green salad with red tomatoes and steamed broccoli. The 40% of the plate to be filled with protein might be dedicated to sliced white turkey meat.

By the way, don't be intimidated by the preciseness of the percentages. You can interpret 60% as a little more than half and 40% as a little less than half. Once you estimate the measurements right, there's no rule against spreading the turkey over the salad greens and calling it a turkey salad.

Snacks? Of course.

Letting yourself get too hungry between meals is counterproductive to your weight-loss efforts. You'll simply be tempted to overeat when mealtime comes.

That's why the Sonoma Diet allows snacking. But like most things, snacking is more restricted during Wave 1 than it is for the rest of the diet.

Between lunch and dinner, or between breakfast and lunch, you may have a small snack to tide you over. When you get to Wave 2, there will be plenty of possibilities. On Wave 1 there is one—a Tier 1 vegetable.

We allow an exception. If you're a bigger man, or if you are a woman or man who leads a very physically active life with plenty of exercise, you can expand your snack menu a bit. Here are some possibilities:

- 115 g/4 oz low-fat cottage cheese with Tier 1 raw veggies
- 85 g/3 oz hummus, either homemade or store-bought, with veggies
- Low-fat cheese stick with carrots or celery
- 1 slice of whole grain bread with one tablespoon of peanut butter
- 50 g/2 oz cooked chicken breast or turkey deli meat

When you reach Wave 2, those choices and many others will be available. For now, though, most should try to keep snacking quick and simple—try a cup of raw pepper strips, some raw broccoli, or a sliced tomato with dried basil and other herbs.

Because you chose the 60–40 ratio for your lunch, the charts tell us that your dinner plate will be filled with 30% protein, 20% grains, and 50% Tier 1 vegetables. How about roasted vegetables on half of your plate, wild rice on 20%, and a grilled 115 g/4 oz cut of lean beef tenderloin for the 30% protein?

What About Fat?

There are no percentages of the plate designated for added fats. Instead, you have three servings of fat a day allotted to use as you see fit. A fat serving is a teaspoon of olive oil, 11 almonds, 14 peanuts, 10 pecan halves, or 7 walnut halves.

A possible use of fats for one day might be a teaspoon of extra-virgin olive oil drizzled over a spinach salad, another teaspoon of olive oil per serving of roast vegetables, and some almonds sprinkled over the salad or as a snack.

Choose or Follow

At the beginning of the recipe section, on page 160, you'll find a meal guide that offers exact food choices for each part of your plate and for every meal throughout the 10-day Wave 1. This has the obvious advantage of taking the guesswork out of the process. You're also guaranteed to eat delicious and healthy meals perfectly planned for weight loss. Each recommendation refers you to a Sonoma-inspired recipe in the book for bringing it to your plate.

You're not obligated to follow this meal guide. If you prefer to pick and choose your own meals according to your own taste, please do so. As long as you stick to the percentages and choose foods appropriate for Wave 1, you'll be eating the Sonoma Diet way. And you'll notice weight loss right away.

That's it. Enjoy. Your Sonoma Diet has now begun.

An Added Boost

It's hard to get all of the nutrients you need in one day on any diet, but especially on a weight-loss plan. That's why you may choose to take one multivitamin a day. You may also want to take a 500 mg calcium supplement. Talk to your doctor about your specific needs.

WAVE 1

Sonoma Tier 1 Vegetables

Unlimited

Asparagus
Aubergine, cooked
Bagged Salad Blend – any type
Bamboo Shoot
Bean, Green
Broccoli, raw or cooked
Brussels Sprouts, cooked
Cabbage, raw or cooked
Cauliflower, raw or cooked
Celery
Chinese Leaves
Courgette
Cucumber
Fennel
Jicama
Kale, cooked
Kohlrabi
Leek, cooked
Lettuce and Leaves – Cos, Beetroot
  Green, Mustard Green,
  Turnip Green, Swiss Chard,
  Kale or other dark green leaf,
  Amaranth, Rocket, Celtuce,
  Endive
Mangetout Pea
Mushroom, raw or cooked
Okra, cooked
Onion, raw or cooked
Pak Choi
Pepper, Yellow, Red, or Green
Radicchio
Radish
Spinach, raw or cooked
Spring Onion
Sprouts – Alfalfa, Kidney Bean,
  Mung Bean
Squash, cooked
Sugar Snap Pea
Tomato, raw
Watercress

Sonoma Proteins and Dairy

PROTEIN

Beans/Legumes – Limit to
  50 g/2 oz per day in Wave 1,
  Chickpea, Black Bean, Pinto
  Bean, Black-Eyed Pea, Lentil,
  Soya Bean (Edamame, Tofu)
Beef
Lean Cuts – Chuck, Fillet, Rump,
  Sirloin
Eggs – 1 whole egg = 2 whites
Fish
Lean: Cod, Flounder, Halibut,
  Perch, Grouper, Pike,
  Monkfish, Haddock, Orange
  Roughy
Moderate-Fat: Striped Bass, Catfish,
  Swordfish, Tuna, Sea Bass,
  Snapper, Whitefish
Higher-Fat: Mackerel, Salmon,
  Trout
Game Meats – Venison
Lamb – Leg, Shank, Fillet,
  Loin, Shoulder
Peanut Butter – 2 tablespoons/
  for main-dish protein,
  1 tablespoon if used as a snack
Pork
Lean Cuts – Ham, boiled or cured;
  Canned Ham; Prosciutto; Fillet;
  Tenderloin; Loin Chop;
  Loin

Poultry – White Meat, no skin;
   Turkey Bacon; Turkey Sausage
Shellfish – Clam, Crab, Lobster,
   Mussel, Oyster, Scallop, Prawn
Soya Substitutes – Vegetarian (Soya)
   Crumble, Vegetarian (Soya) Burger
Veal – Minced, Leg, Fillet, Loin,
   Shoulder

DAIRY

Fat-Free Skimmed Milk, up to
   225 ml/8 fl oz on cereal for
   breakfast only
Low-Fat Cottage Cheese
Low-Fat Cheese – Grated
   Parmesan, Mozzarella – 25 g/1 oz

Sonoma Grains

70 g/2½ oz = 1 serving
Barley, cooked
Brown, Red, or Black Rice, cooked
Bulgur, cooked
Oats – Pinhead Oatmeal,
   Rolled Oats, Oat Bran
Popcorn, air-popped, no butter*
Quinoa, cooked
Soba Noodle, cooked
Wheat – Cracked Wheat; Bulgur;
   Wheat Berry, cooked
Whole Grain Bread, 1 slice (2 or
   more grams fibre per slice)
Whole Grain Cereal, 8 grams fibre
   per serving or higher
Whole Grain Pasta, cooked
Wild Rice

* intended for a snack, not to go on the plate

Beverages

Black, Green, or Herbal Tea, no
   cream or sugar
Coffee, black or with up to 2 packets
   artificial sweetener and maximum
   1 tablespoon heavy cream
Water, plain or sparkling

Sonoma Fats

**Up to 3 servings per day
one teaspoon = 1 serving**
Olive Oil
Avocado – ¼

Nuts
Almonds – 11
Peanuts – 14
Pecans – 10 halves
Walnuts – 7 halves

Flavour Boosters

Unlimited
Herbs – Basil, Coriander, Chives, Dill,
   Fennel, Marjoram, Mint, Oregano,
   Rosemary, Sage, Tarragon, Thyme
Spices – Caraway, Cardamom,
   Cayenne, Celery Seed, Chilli
   Powder, Cinnamon, Clove,
   Cumin, Curry, Nutmeg, Pepper,
   Saffron, Turmeric
Chilli Pepper
Garlic
Ginger
Horseradish
Lemon or Lime Juice or Zest
Lemongrass
Mustard (all types)
Vanilla
Vinegar – Rice Wine, Balsamic

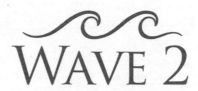

WAVE 2

Welcome to Wave 2, the major part of your diet. This is the eating plan you'll stay with until you reach your target weight. It's the meat and potatoes of the diet—without the potatoes.

While Wave 1 helped you through a transition period of rapid weight loss, Wave 2 keeps the weight loss going. The loss isn't as fast as in Wave 1, but it's steady, healthy, and noticeable. It's the kind of weight loss that lasts a lifetime.

With Wave 2 comes your full enjoyment of the Sonoma Diet lifestyle. That means pleasurable eating, a heightened appreciation of fresh, wholesome foods, and a new, energetic physical health you can feel all day long. So it's very important that you continue to make at least one daily meal a long and leisurely affair where you take your time to savour every bite. And keep with whatever exercise you've chosen to do (see "Fast-Track Your Weight Loss" beginning on page 94).

More than anything else, Wave 2 is about variety. We've been driving home the variety message since the beginning of this book—not just for the extra zest it brings to meals but also for its role in health and weight loss. Now you'll take variety to the next level. Your food choices multiply significantly in Wave 2, and so do the suggested recipes.

All the Top Ten Power Foods introduced earlier in the book are now available to you. Fruits have returned to your daily diet. Two new "tiers" of vegetables join the line-up as well. You now have scores of fruits and vegetables to choose from, and you'll be encouraged to eat plenty of them.

Fat-free yogurt (plain) is a new dairy choice. You're allowed some sugar-free desserts, if you still want them. Maybe even a piece of dark chocolate on occasion. Honey is back in too and will prove particularly useful for sweetening up some of the Sonoma Diet recipes. A glass of wine can now be part of one of your daily meals. Snacks, too, can be a little more varied and substantive.

The grains list stays the same on Wave 2, because it already includes most of the whole grains you'll be able to find easily. Your fat allotment remains at three servings a day in the form of extra-virgin olive oil, walnuts, almonds, peanuts, pecans, and avocados. (Remember, though, that these are in addition to the fats found in your protein sources and other foods.)

All in all, you'll find Wave 2 much easier than Wave 1. That's because it's designed for the long haul. Plus there's that big boost in variety. Extra satisfaction and extra variety make for a pretty good one-two punch for your confidence. And it's very much in keeping with the Sonoma Diet approach of achieving weight loss by eating pleasing portions of delicious, healthy foods.

You may reach your target weight in a few weeks, a few months, or longer. No two dieters have the same task. But because of its emphasis on rich flavours and nutrient-rich meals, Wave 2 should never feel like drudgery or sacrifice, no matter how long it takes. Think of it as new adventures in eating rather than a diet. The pounds will vanish either way.

YOUR WAVE 2 EATING GUIDE

The instructions for Wave 2 are even simpler than Wave 1. You don't have to overhaul your kitchen again, but do stock up on some of the new fruits and vegetables you're now encouraged to eat.

And, oh yes, choose a few bottles of decent, modestly priced wine. Invest in one of those handpump/plastic stopper set-ups so you can save what you don't drink. (It'll keep just fine that way for a few days.)

You'll be using exactly the same plates and bowls. As you look at the plate

Breakfast

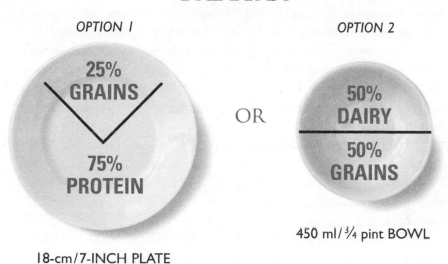

OPTION 1

25%
GRAINS

75%
PROTEIN

OR

OPTION 2

50%
DAIRY

50%
GRAINS

450 ml / ¾ pint BOWL

18-cm / 7-INCH PLATE

Lunch and Dinner

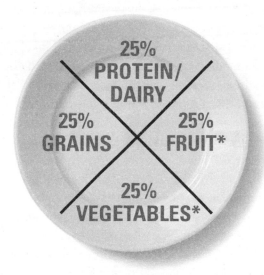

25%
PROTEIN/
DAIRY

25%
GRAINS

25%
FRUIT*

25%
VEGETABLES*

23-cm / 9-INCH PLATE

* CHOOSE FROM TIERS 1, 2, OR 3.

illustrations, you'll see that your breakfast options are basically the same. But there's another choice (not illustrated on page 79)—a bowl of pure dairy. What that essentially comes down to is a breakfast of plain low-fat yogurt. That's a great option if you love yogurt. Otherwise, you'll want to go with the milk-and-cereal choice, or the 75% protein plate (with 25% grains, probably as a piece of whole grain bread or toast), or the 100% protein option. The protein plate, of course, offers the most possibilities. Remember that eggs go with protein, not dairy.

For lunch and dinner, you'll use the same plate proportions, though you'll want to choose different foods. You're really just dividing your plate into four parts and filling one part with grains, one with vegetables, one with fruit, and one with either a protein choice or dairy (which might be low-fat cheese or cottage cheese).

That's it. Use your same three fat allotments as in Wave 1—a sprinkling of nuts or a little olive oil either to cook with or to wake up greens or other vegetables as part of a dressing.

There are plenty of recipes to guide you. Remember that the tastiest and most beneficial food combinations are built into these recipes, so take advantage of them.

You also have the option of following the food guide, which tells you exactly what to have at each meal. The guide will take you through two weeks of different meal plans. If that two-week stretch doesn't get you to your target weight (and it probably won't unless you were just a tad overweight to start with), simply run through the cycle again.

THE FIBRE CONNECTION

There's another reason Wave 2 will seem easier. By now you've reduced your cravings for sugar and refined white flour. You may have even eliminated those cravings completely. If you haven't, don't despair. You will soon.

Using Wave 1 to get rid of the white bread and sweets habit will pay big dividends in Wave 2. And make no mistake about it, "habit" is the right way to put it. Is there a better word to describe your daily chocolate bar and soft drink from the vending machine? Or the bag of cracker-like treats that disappears while you're watching television or riding the bus?

In Wave 2, you continue to ban refined sugar from your diet. Now, however, you can replace it with sweet power fruits such as blueberries and strawberries. You've already replaced white flour products with whole grains. Those two substitutions alone are a big part of what makes Wave 2 work.

But the most relevant benefit of these two smart switches is their effect on your metabolism, or the way your system processes food as potential energy. To repeat, sugar and refined flour convert to blood sugar (glucose) and then to body fat very quickly. Whole grains and most fruits and vegetables go through the digestion process more slowly and are less likely to be converted to body fat. Fibre is the major reason for this difference. Eating fibre-rich foods is also a natural way to curb hunger. Over time, you notice the benefits of the slower pace when you stand on your bathroom scales.

Fibre in Your Favour

Fibre is most abundant in whole grains, legumes, vegetables, and fruits. Not coincidentally, those are staples of the Sonoma Diet. Fibre's mere presence is why you can eat so many fruits and vegetables in Wave 2 even though they do contain natural sugars. Fibre's presence is also why whole grains are acceptable while fibre-depleted refined grains are taboo.

There are actually two kinds of dietary fibre. One dissolves in water; the other doesn't. Generally speaking (and with some key exceptions), whole grains and vegetables contain insoluble fibre. Nuts, seeds, legumes, and fruits contain soluble fibre.

For your weight-loss purposes, this is mostly a distinction without a difference. Each kind of fibre helps slow blood sugar release. And because you'll be eating plant foods in an abundant variety, you'll get plenty of both in Wave 2 anyway.

Which puts you well ahead of the majority of people, who get about half the amount of fibre they need each day. Remember to make sure that every slice of whole grain bread you eat has at least 2 grams of fibre in it and that every bowl of whole grain cereal has at least 8 grams of fibre.

Fibre for Health

As with just about anything you eat on the Sonoma Diet, fibre works complementarily as a weight-loss aid and health protector. There's an obvious link between high-fibre diets and diabetes prevention because diabetes is characterized by an inability to properly process blood sugar levels. Not only does weight loss itself lower your diabetes risk, there's also evidence that diets rich in high-fibre whole grains also reduce your chances of getting it.

As the Mediterraneans show us, fibre is protective against heart disease. According to a Harvard study of 40,000 subjects, eating lots of fibre is associated with a 40% lower heart disease risk compared to low fibre intake.

Soluble fibres especially lower blood cholesterol levels. That's one reason why porridge is such a fine breakfast choice; it's one of the few grains with more soluble than unsoluble fibre, so it's simultaneously an effective cholesterol lowerer, digestion slower, and energy booster.

And don't overlook fibre's gastrointestinal benefits. It helps you avoid intestinal inflammation and is well-known for its ability to relieve or prevent constipation. Again, grain fibre, especially wheat bran and oat bran, seems to work the best. But a high-fibre diet in general is the surest way to get all these health benefits.

Going Glycaemic

Naturally, not all plant foods have the same amount or type of fibre. Nor do they have the same amount or type of sugar. So different fruits, vegetables, grains, and other plant foods boost blood sugar at different speeds and in different amounts.

Nutritionists have come up with a way of measuring those rates. It's called the Glycaemic Index. Basically, it assigns white bread the arbitrary number of 100 and measures every other plant food against it. The higher the number, the faster the food shoots your blood sugar levels up. And then the faster they get pushed too far down as insulin pours in to deal with the sugar.

Foods with the lower Glycaemic Index (or GI) rating metabolize more slowly, turn to body fat less readily, and may satisfy your hunger longer. A baked potato, for example, has a high GI number—typically reported at 85. Spinach and broccoli have a number under 0. Guess which one isn't on the Sonoma Diet food list and which are Top Ten Sonoma Diet Power Foods?

For the most part, high GI foods are to be avoided—such as white bread (GI of 100), refined commercial cereals (mostly in the 80 to 120 range), and sugars (mostly from 80 to 150). The low GI foods are usually preferred.

But as useful as the Glycaemic Index can be, you don't need to deal with it on the Sonoma Diet. For one thing, we don't believe that numbers and enjoyable eating go together. From the beginning, we've spared you calorie counts, protein gram counts, carbohydrate gram counts, fat gram counts, and food portion weights. We're certainly not going to burden you with a number to assign to most of the foods you put on your plate.

Besides, the Glycaemic Index can be confusing and misleading. The numbers themselves tend to change depending on where you find them. And they're often irrelevant. For example, although whole grains have lower GI numbers, a slice of whole grain bread might have roughly the same GI number as a slice of white bread. But they're certainly not equivalent—for your health, for your metabolism, for your weight loss.

Also, a commercial chocolate bar with peanuts may have a fairly low GI number. Load sugar up with enough saturated fat and, yes, it will release more slowly in your bloodstream. That doesn't make it a good choice for somebody trying to lose weight—or anybody trying to stay healthy, for that matter.

So we'll stick to the Sonoma Diet way of doing things. We've done the thinking, measuring, and ranking of all the foods for you. Your only job is to pick your favourites, put the right amounts on your plate, and enjoy. Leave the statistics to the sports pages.

Mix and Match

Food partnering for maximum health and taste as well as quicker weight loss defines the Sonoma Diet. Extra-virgin olive oil is such an important food on the diet, not just because of its heart-healthy action but also because of its unique (among oils) ability to add and bring out the nutrients and flavour of other foods. With cooked tomatoes, it helps your body absorb more of the disease-preventing lycopenes. With spinach and other dark leafy greens, it brings out the phytonutrients while mellowing that hint of bitterness in the leaves.

So when you see unfamiliar foods or food combinations in the recipes, rest assured that they're there for a reason. Much planning has gone into the mixes and matches to bring out the maximum benefits. From something as simple as nuts over a salad to more involved plans such as mixing lean beef and a citrus vinaigrette into a vegetable stir-fry, all of it's the result of expert nutritionists at work with your weight loss in mind.

Combos are the main reason to ignore the Glycaemic Index: it's based on foods in isolation, whereas we usually eat them combined with other foods. How you combine foods shifts the GI number.

Take the whole grain pasta you'll probably be enjoying from time to time. It doesn't have all that high a GI number to start with. But the number goes down sharply when it's prepared according to the Sonoma Diet recipes. So pasta provides a clear case in point of the Sonoma Diet approach to health and weight loss. A problem food—pasta—turns into a healthy weight-loss food when you 1) eat the whole grain version, 2) prepare it with other ingredients that slow its blood sugar release, 3) limit the use of saturated fats such as those found in high-fat cheeses by using low-fat cheeses such as Parmesan and mozzarella instead, and 4) eat it slowly in reasonable portions.

FRUITS ARE BACK

One of the biggest sacrifices you had to make during Wave 1 was going without fruit for 10 days. It was all about the sugar. One reason fruits taste so great is their sugar content, in the form of fructose. Fructose is the most benign sugar there is, with a slow release in the bloodstream and without adverse effects.

But sugar is sugar. And forcing yourself off the sugar bandwagon was so high a priority in Wave 1 that we didn't even want you eating foods that reminded you of sugar. Ten days without fruits' health and weight-loss properties was a stiff price to pay, we know, but worth it to help break the sugar habit. Until you're off the sugar-and-white-flour merry-go-round, you'll never reach your weight goal or be truly healthy.

And look at it this way: "Low-carb" diets discourage fruits for life, and some even outright ban them. You're way ahead of the game.

You'll be eating two fruit servings a day on Wave 2. For typically sized fruits (apples, oranges, peaches, etc.), a serving is about one fruit. For bigger fruits such as papayas and pineapples, and for smaller berries and grapes and the like, a serving is 70 g/2½ oz.

There are two tiers of fruits, based on their content of calories and natural sugars. Because there were no fruits in Wave 1 of the diet, there are not Tier 1 fruits. Instead, fruits are found in Tiers 2 and 3. You may choose both your daily servings from this group. Tier 3 fruits (such as bananas, figs, mangoes, and peaches) have more sugar and/or less water, so there are fewer nutrients per calorie. One of your daily servings can come from this group, but the other must come from Tier 2.

The Lure of Fruits

As you know, blueberries, strawberries, and grapes make our Top Ten Sonoma Diet Power Food list. They're also examples of how the fruit on your dinner plate can serve as dessert. Though those three take top honours, they're hardly alone among power fruits. Each fruit on the Sonoma Diet Fruits lists has its own health-imparting chemical make-up, and most have it in amounts that rival the Top Ten Power Foods. Most are heart protective.

One point to remember is the synergistic nature of each fruit's nutrients—that is, how they work together to strengthen your heart and otherwise make you healthier. That's why buying whole, fresh, ripe fruits is ideal. You want to get every ounce of benefit from what you eat.

Apples: A Power Food Alternative

Use apples as an alternative Top Ten Sonoma Diet Power Food. When you bite into a cool, crisp apple, you're treating yourself to a cornucopia of disease-fighting antioxidants. Among fruits, only berries and prunes have more. You're also getting a double dose of fibre, the undigested part of plant carbohydrates that eases waste and toxins out of your body. A typical apple will deliver at least 3 grams of fibre.

Drinking fruit juices, as we mentioned before, is not a good idea. Commercial juices have usually had nutrients processed out of them and sugar added into them. Even the better fresh-squeezed juices compromise the "power food" concept of the Sonoma Diet. You get no feeling of "eating satisfaction" from drinking juice. You're not chewing anything. So juice usually ends up as added-on calories. That slows down your weight loss.

Be careful with canned fruits. They almost always have added sugar, which is a no-no. They're also often peeled or otherwise diminished. Stick to fresh fruits from the market. Fruits that freeze well, however, such as berries, can be bought frozen.

We won't run through the phytonutrients of all the fruits you're now encouraged to eat. You got a pretty good idea of the power of the special nutrients that fruits contain when we described blueberries, strawberries, and grapes in the Sonoma Diet Power Foods chapter.

Your Vegetable Bin Grows

With Wave 2, the full panoply of vegetables we reviewed in the last chapter is now available to you. In addition to the Tier 1 vegetables you ate in Wave 1, you now have Tier 2 and Tier 3 vegetables.

Again, the higher tiers simply reflect a higher sugar and calorie level. At the highest tier (Tier 3) you'll find squashes, peas, sweetcorn, and sweet potatoes. These are fine vegetables, but make sure you choose only one serving a day from this list. And remember, one serving is not necessarily an entire yam. It's about 85 g/3 oz, cooked and sliced or wedged.

During Wave 2, choose one Tier 2 vegetable and one Tier 3 vegetable per day. Remember, as in Wave 1, you can still enjoy unlimited amounts of the Tier 1 vegetables throughout the day with meals or as snacks.

Wave 2 Desserts

If you still crave desserts, don't have any. That may sound backwards, but eliminating those cravings is still your goal. Now that you're on Wave 2, you have the option of satisfying your sweet tooth with such fruits as berries or mangoes. You'll be surprised at how satisfyingly sweet they can be. Fruit is your dessert of choice. Try using your lunch and/or dinner fruit serving (25% of the plate) to satisfy that end-of-meal-sweet desire.

For those who absolutely must have a special dessert-type treat, try dark, bittersweet chocolate. It's allowed in small amounts as occasional treats—one bite-size piece a day, no more than three days a week.

A LITTLE WINE WITH THAT?

When you think about a family in southern France or Italy sitting down to a meal, you assume there's wine on the table. That's the Mediterranean way.

It's the Sonoma way as well. Sonoma County and neighbouring Napa County comprise one of the most important winemaking regions in the world. Locally grown wine is a way of life in Sonoma as much as in France, Spain, or Italy. It's a fixture on the dinner table.

Wine was put on hold during Wave 1, partly for the sugar and partly because Wave 1 was more calorie-stingy than Wave 2. But that's over now. Wave 2 is wine time.

From now on, you are encouraged to accompany one daily meal (presumably dinner) with a glass of red or white wine. We say "encouraged" rather than "allowed" because moderate wine consumption delivers health benefits perfectly in keeping with the Sonoma Diet philosophy. For a modest amount of calories, a daily glass of wine has been clearly shown in recent years to reduce your risk of heart disease. There is hardly any doubt left about this among cardiologists and nutritionists.

At the same time, wine imparts a mealtime sense of relaxation and enjoyment that is so essential to your new weight-loss lifestyle. Besides the obvious gustatory delight that a good glass of wine adds to food enjoyment, the very act of choosing wine, opening it, pouring it, and drinking it slows down the whole eating process—which is just what you want.

The wine ritual focuses attention on the sensuality of the occasion and away from any over-eagerness to simply stuff food in your mouth. Wine reminds us that mealtime is about pleasure, not just filling up. Savour the wine and taste the food. You reawaken senses and food experiences that perhaps have been forgotten. You're satisfied with less and eat slower. You lose weight and gain insight on how to eat for pleasure.

Note, though, that the word "obligated" wasn't used about wine either. If there's any medical or health reason why you shouldn't drink wine, by all means don't touch it. If you don't like wine, don't drink it. If you give it a try with a little help from a wine-loving friend and still don't like it, don't drink it.

But if you're used to enjoying wine, make it a part of one daily meal. Keep it to one glass and make it last. Wine isn't there to quench your thirst. It's there to enhance your experience.

Wine and Your Health

There's plenty of evidence that alcohol itself, in moderation, has cardiovascular benefits. But wine's heart-protective effect goes beyond the alcohol. It's the result of a huge array of phytonutrients, including flavonoids and most notably an amazing compound called resveratrol. You met resveratrol when we introduced table grapes as a power food. Its heart-protective antioxidant action is even stronger in wine than in grapes.

Because of these special nutrients, many scientific studies have concluded that wine consumption is much more strongly correlated with reduced risk of death from heart disease than drinking alcohol in general. In these studies, "moderate consumption" is defined as 1 to 3 drinks per day. Of course, we're on a tight budget when it comes to calories, so follow the one

---

Wave 2 Snacks

Snacks are to keep you from being uncomfortably hungry between meals. The best choice is still a Tier 1 vegetable, prepared however you like it. The trick with snacking between meals is to walk the line—you want to calm hunger so you won't be starving come mealtime. But you don't want to use that as an excuse to overeat, slowing down your weight-loss progress.

But now that you're on Wave 2, you have more choices—if you need them. Some of the following will look familiar; they were permitted to men and physically active women in Wave 1.

- A Tier 2 fruit, keeping to the 70 g/2½ oz serving size.
- A spoonful or two of low-fat cottage cheese with a little sliced Tier 2 fruit.
- Half a bag of light microwave-popped popcorn. Plain—no oil or butter.
- A piece of mozzarella cheese or a slice of lean cooked meat.
- 115 g/4 oz low-fat cottage cheese with Tier 1 raw veggies
- 85 g/3 oz hummus, either homemade or store-bought, with veggies
- Low-fat cheese stick with carrots or celery
- 1 slice of whole grain bread with 1 tablespoon of peanut butter
- 50 g/2 oz cooked chicken breast or turkey deli meat
- A piece of chicken breast
- One serving of nuts (remember, you've used up a fat serving this way)

---

170 ml/6 fl oz glass per day guideline during Wave 2.

There's even good reason to believe that wine has much to do with the lower rates of heart disease in southern Europe. Here's why. Not everybody in all parts of the countries touching the Mediterranean follows the Mediterranean diet. Many have simply succumbed to the bad dietary habits of much of the Western world. But in France, for example, even those people who eat higher-fat diets still get less heart disease than other westerners.

This curiosity was dubbed the French Paradox. And the explanation has to

---

The Sonoma Diet Wine 101

Enjoying wine doesn't require a degree in winemaking. Good wine is wine you enjoy drinking. Period. Try different varieties to figure out what types of wine are appealing to you and experiment by drinking different wines with foods to find combinations you enjoy. You've already learned about smart food combinations for health and flavour—such as a fresh squeeze of lemon juice on seafood or a drizzle of olive oil over your dark leafy greens. Wine plays a similar role by enhancing these flavours in food. In general, pair light-bodied wines with lighter foods that use delicate preparations. Full-bodied wines go better with heartier, more intense flavours. Your Wave 2 meal plans offer some recommendations for a variety of wines to accompany your evening meals. Here are some ideas for pairing wine with food:

WHITE WINES
- Chardonnay: seafood, chicken, ham, veal
- Sauvignon Blanc: oysters, salmon, goat's cheese, salads, pasta
- Riesling: mild cheeses, pork, tandoori chicken, shellfish
- Sparkling white wines: Asian, Thai, curry, chilli pepper spices

RED WINES
- Cabernet Sauvignon: duck, spicy beef and poultry, richer foods in general
- Pinot Noir: braised chicken, turkey, lamb, mushrooms, earthy flavours
- Merlot: braised chicken, roasted beef, lamb, game
- Burgundy: salmon, tuna, roast chicken
- Chianti: pasta with tomato sauce, pizza

---

do with wine. It was eventually determined that regular wine consumption provides protection against heart disease even for folks who consider butter an appetizer. Combine regular, moderate wine drinking with a better, Mediterranean-style diet, and you have a formula for health.

Several Harvard University studies have been collecting information regarding the building blocks for a healthy lifestyle. The researchers have found common habits for better health. People who have these lifestyle habits had 80% fewer heart attacks and more than 90% fewer cases of diabetes than other subjects. The top five traits or habits are avoid obesity, consume a healthy diet, avoid smoking, engage in moderate physical activity, and drink ½ to 2 servings of an alcoholic beverage—such as wine—each day.

The Sonoma Diet includes wine as a component of one of your daily meals. Since many of the beneficial effects of wine are transient—meaning they last about 24 hours—the best pattern is to drink moderately each day, rather than saving your weekly wine allotment for the weekend. Also, recent studies show that when wine is consumed with food there are favourable effects on the body's absorption of antioxidants from the food and wine, as well as the metabolism of dietary fats in the body.

That's what the Sonoma Diet does. Is it any wonder we like the idea of a glass of wine at dinner?

WAVE 2

Sonoma Tier 1
Vegetables

Unlimited, see Wave 1 listing

Sonoma Tier 2
Fruits & Vegetables

**Limit to 1 fruit and 1 vegetable from
this list per day**
**70 g/2½ oz = 1 serving or 1 whole
small piece of fruit**

FRUITS
Apple
Apricot
Blackberry
Blueberry
Boysenberry
Cantaloupe
Cherry – sour only
Gooseberry, raw
Grape
Grapefruit
Honeydew Melon
Huckleberry
Kiwifruit
Kumquat
Lemon
Lime
Mulberry
Orange
Papaya
Pineapple
Plum
Pomelo (Chinese Grapefruit)
Quince
Raspberry
Rhubarb
Starfruit
Strawberry
Tangerine
Ugli Fruit
Watermelon

VEGETABLES
Artichoke
Beetroot, cooked
Carrot, raw or cooked
Celeriac, raw or cooked
Chilli Pepper
Jerusalem Artichoke
Pumpkin, raw or cooked
Spaghetti Squash
Swede, cooked
Water Chestnut

Sonoma Tier 3
Fruits & Vegetables

**Limit to 1 fruit and 1 vegetable from
this list per day**
**70 g/2½ oz = 1 serving or 1 whole
small piece of fruit**

FRUIT
Banana
Elderberry
Fig
Guava
Mango
Nectarine
Passion Fruit
Peach
Pear
Persimmon
Plantain
Pomegranate

VEGETABLES

Acorn Squash
Butternut Squash
Mangetout pea, raw or cooked
Parsnip
Pea, cooked
Sugar Snap Pea
Sweetcorn
Sweet Potato, cooked
Yam

Sonoma Proteins and Dairy

PROTEIN

Beans/Legumes – Chickpea, Black
   Bean, Pinto Bean, Black-Eyed Pea,
   Lentil, Soya Bean (Edamame, Tofu)
Beef
Lean Cuts – Chuck, Fillet, Rump,
   Sirloin
Eggs – 1 whole egg = 2 whites
Fish
Lean: Cod, Flounder, Halibut,
   Perch, Grouper, Pike,
   Monkfish, Haddock, Orange
   Roughy
Moderate-Fat: Striped Bass, Catfish,
   Swordfish, Tuna, Sea Bass,
   Snapper, Whitefish
Higher-Fat: Mackerel, Salmon,
   Trout
Game Meats – Venison
Lamb – Leg, Shank, Fillet, Loin,
   Shoulder
Peanut Butter – 2 tablespoons
   for main-dish protein,
   1 tablespoon if used as a snack
Pork
Lean Cuts – Ham, boiled or cured;
   Canned Ham; Prosciutto; Fillet;
   Tenderloin; Loin Chop; Loin
Poultry – White Meat, no skin;
   Turkey Bacon; Turkey Sausage
Shellfish – Clam, Crab, Lobster,
   Mussel, Oyster, Scallop, Prawn
Soya Substitutes – Vegetarian
   (Soya) Crumble, Vegetarian (Soya)
   Burger
Veal – Minced, Leg, Fillet, Loin,
   Shoulder

DAIRY

Fat-Free Plain Yogurt, 225 g/8 oz
Fat-Free Skimmed Milk,
   225 ml/8 fl oz
Low-Fat Cottage Cheese
Low-Fat Cheese – Grated
   Parmesan, Mozzarella – 25 g/1 oz

Sonoma Grains

70 g/2½ oz = 1 serving
Barley, cooked
Brown, Red, or Black Rice, cooked
Bulgur, cooked
Oats – Pinhead Oatmeal,
   Rolled Oats, Oat Bran
Popcorn, air-popped, no butter*
Quinoa, cooked
Soba Noodle, cooked
Wheat – Cracked Wheat; Bulgur;
   Wheat Berry, cooked
Whole Grain Bread, 1 slice (2 or
   more grams fibre per slice)
Whole Grain Cereal, 8 grams fibre
   per serving or higher
Whole Grain Pasta, cooked
Wild Rice

* *intended for a snack, not to go on the plate*

Beverages

Black, Green, or Herbal Tea, no
cream or sugar
Coffee, black or with up to 2 packets
artificial sweetener and maximum
1 tablespoon heavy cream
Water, plain or sparkling
Wine (Red or White) – 170 ml/6 fl oz
per day

Lemon or Lime Juice or Zest
Lemongrass
Mustard (all types)
Vanilla
Vinegar – Rice Wine, Balsamic

Sonoma Fats

**Up to 3 servings per day
one teaspoon = 1 serving**

Olive Oil
Avocado – ¼

Nuts
Almonds – 11
Peanuts – 14
Pecans – 10 halves
Walnuts – 7 halves

Flavour Boosters

Unlimited
Herbs – Basil, Coriander, Chives, Dill,
Fennel, Marjoram, Mint, Oregano,
Rosemary, Sage, Tarragon, Thyme
Spices – Caraway, Cardamom,
Cayenne, Celery Seed, Chilli
Powder, Cinnamon, Clove,
Cumin, Curry, Nutmeg, Pepper,
Saffron, Turmeric
Chilli Pepper
Garlic
Ginger
Horseradish

FAST-TRACK YOUR WEIGHT LOSS

The Sonoma Diet has an especially outstanding advantage: it's easier to stick to because the meal plans and recipes are designed for pleasure. Because you're eating better than you were before, there's less temptation to go back to the bad old ways.

But there's also a disadvantage, one that's common to all diets. The disadvantage is that the Sonoma Diet takes place in the real world. And in the real world, nothing is easy all the time.

In the real world, you can get impatient at what seems like too slow a weight-loss pace. You can understand the diet rules down to the last detail but still find them hard to follow. Or you may sense your enthusiasm slipping away, making you a candidate for the diet blues.

Even worse, cravings lurk in the real world. So do lapses, temptations, and mistakes. Incidents occur, sometimes involving entire pints of ice cream. Frustration might set in. Seemingly for no reason, you hit plateaus where a week or more goes by without an ounce of weight lost.

And sometimes, well, you just don't care how good the Sonoma Diet food is. You want bad food, you want a lot of it, and you want it right now.

Sound familiar? All of these distractions are to be expected. They are totally normal. That's why it's called the "real world."

The first five chapters of this book explained to you what to do and why you're doing it. In this chapter, we'll tell you how to do it—and how to keep on doing it when times get tough. You'll see that the real-world problems are part and parcel of any diet and that there are simple ways to overcome any rough patch you stumble across on the road to your ideal weight.

Make no mistake about it; you will get past the pitfalls, great or small. Your body wants to be at its best weight. All you're doing is helping it along.

You're Not Alone

The first thing to realize is that everybody struggles at times with any diet. Everybody fights cravings. Everybody gives into temptation once in a while. And everybody goes through periods when he or she feels like giving up.

You're not alone. Others have been through exactly what you're going through. And they came out the other side slimmer, healthier, and happier.

What's happening is that your body and mind are resisting change. It doesn't matter that the change is for the better or that it mostly feels good. It's still change, and your brain is hardwired to resist change. Or at least to be very cautious about accepting it.

Think about how many new habits you've been adopting. You're eating less. You're eating more slowly. You're eating healthier foods in a greater variety. You've kicked what was probably a lifelong habit of loading up on refined flour and sugar. You've changed the kind of dietary fat you're consuming.

Your body thanks you every day for these changes. At the same time, though, your brain is wondering what happened to all that other stuff you used to love so much. Occasionally it will remind you about them.

That's what cravings and temptations are—reminders of change. They're just thoughts. And you can deal with thoughts.

Get Things Out in the Open

The way to deal with those thoughts is openly and directly. Cravings and other diet pitfalls aren't vague annoyances that might go away. They are specific reactions to specific situations. So they can be isolated, confronted, and understood. That's what you need to do to get them to go away.

It will help you get a handle on things to remember that lapses are really part of the diet. They're natural by-products of any eating regimen change. And they've been taken into consideration from the earliest planning stages.

In other words, the Sonoma Diet was designed with the full understanding that anyone who follows it is going to deviate from the guidelines on occasion. It's expected. So when you give into a craving, or eat too much of the wrong thing, we've got you covered.

Say you get invited to a dinner party and end up finishing a plate of fatty prime rib with a baked potato drenched with soured cream and butter. Obviously, this was not a good idea. But you haven't been weak. You haven't sinned. You haven't gone "off the diet." You're only guilty of behaving like a human being. You had a bad night. Shrug it off and move forward.

Of course, you'll lose weight quicker when these lapses occur less frequently. You'll certainly enjoy the diet more if you're not constantly struggling against cravings and temptations. That's why you're encouraged to deal with these problems as methodically as you do with the eating part of the diet.

Here's what we mean by that: to get down to your target weight, you knew it wouldn't be enough to simply decide to eat a little less or try to cut down on "fattening" foods. Instead, you chose to follow the Sonoma Diet meal plans and eat according to the diet guidelines. It's the same with your cravings. It's not enough to resolve to "be strong" or to wait for them to eventually disappear. You need a plan.

The plan that works is getting the problems out in the open so you can understand where they're coming from and then deal with them. Let's look at the best ways to do that.

Get It Down on Paper

By far the most successful strategy for minimizing problems while sticking to a diet is a food journal. Just the act of writing things down every day serves to focus your attention on eating right.

But a journal does much more than that. Over the weeks it starts to clarify for you the whole confusing interplay of hunger, food, cravings, moods, and all the other things you feel and think and do in the course of a day. Pretty soon, the problems you're having with the diet start making sense.

It's understood that for certain people, keeping a journal—especially a "diet diary"—is unappealing, to put it mildly. Some absolutely detest the idea. If that's you, breathe easy. A food journal is not obligatory on the Sonoma Diet. But bear with us. You need to deal with these things one way or another. A food journal is a proven way to do it.

Quick Tips for Quicker Weight Loss

If you could lose weight even faster than the typical Sonoma Diet pace, would you do it? Here are some simple ways to speed up the process, without sacrificing the health benefits.

• Choose more of your vegetables from Tier 1, retaining just enough Tier 2 and 3 vegetables to maintain variety. Tier 1 vegetables are more nutrient rich, with fewer calories.

• Likewise, choose most of your fruits from Tier 2, leaving Tier 3 fruits for special occasions. Tier 2 fruits have less natural sugar and fewer calories.

• Eat even more slowly. The longer you take at a meal, the less you're likely to eat and the more satisfied you'll feel. Find ways to slow down at all three meals, not just the one very leisurely meal of the day.

• Eat more chicken and fish for protein than red meat, beans, or eggs.

• Skimp on your plate filling. There's no rule saying you have to load it up to the edges. Portions just a tiny bit smaller will pay off over the long run.

• Keep your snacking at Wave 1 level. That means nothing more than a Tier 1 vegetable. If that's enough to tide you over until the next meal, why have more?

• Drink your snack. Try having a cup of hot tea or a tall glass of water instead of your usual snack. You may be more thirsty than hungry, and as long as you're not reaching your next meal in starvation mode, those uneaten calories will pay off.

• Buy food instead of packages. Challenge yourself to buy only fresh food for a week—meat and fish from the butcher, fruit and vegetables from the produce section, whole grains from the health food shop, etc. When you buy "food" instead of "packages," you're eliminating any chance of unwanted processing, refined grains, added hydrogenated fats, and mysterious chemicals sneaking into your diet.

• If you haven't been exercising, start. If you have been exercising, push up the intensity a notch.

It's a tool for losing weight faster and easier. If it works, why not go for it? Every day, write down what you eat, what time you ate it, how much of it you ate, where you were eating it (family table, restaurant, car, desk), and whether you liked it or not. Note how hungry you felt as you began to eat, and what else you were feeling (bored, indifferent, excited). This goes for snacks and meals, as well as whatever little extras find their way into your mouth.

Also jot down throughout the day any thoughts, feelings, or activities worth noting and what time they occurred. Feeling stressed? Write down when and (if you know) why. A special meeting or appointment? Write it down and how you feel about it, before and after. A craving? Write down when and for what.

This may sound like a lot of daylong note taking, but you'll soon create shorthand ways of getting these things down quickly and effortlessly. After all, you're the only one who needs to decipher your scribblings. The main goal, obviously, is to be honest and thorough; you can't deal with your extra snacking if you pretend it's not happening.

After a few days of journal keeping, you can start looking for patterns that might shed some light on some of the problems you've been having with the diet. Do you tend to eat late at night as you watch television? Do you get cravings when you're stressed or bored? Do you often overeat when specific foods are on the plate? Do your cravings seem to come a few hours after certain kinds of meals? Do you yearn for sugar on Mondays?

The connections between cravings and specific moods or habits might be quite clear. Or they might be very subtle. Either way, seeing the patterns demystifies the cravings and makes them much easier to conquer. Trust us.

You'll also find that your food journal will help pin down other reasons you're not losing weight as fast as you'd like. For example, your journal might reveal that you're eating more than you thought you were or that your snacks are regularly too generous. You might see that you're not getting enough variety in your plant foods or protein sources. Maybe you've been eating vegetables from the three tiers in the wrong proportions.

All of this is worth knowing. The knowledge will help you lose weight more quickly and efficiently.

Crave Busters

Magical as it sounds, the very awareness of your craving patterns can itself help you conquer them. Sometimes it's easier to work through a craving when you know it's coming.

But you also might need to take action to keep yourself from falling into the same trap time and again. Much of the time, your course of action is obvious. If you used to mindlessly snack while watching late-night television, don't watch it. It's highly recommended that you don't have meals in front of the TV anyway. Instead, try going to sleep earlier. Studies show getting enough sleep plays a role in weigh loss. If you've realized that you never resist the bagels with cream cheese that your co-workers bring in every Friday morning, make yourself scarce at bagel time. You can't say you weren't warned.

When you feel a craving coming on, take proactive measures. Change the subject in your mind. Go for a walk immediately. Go brush your teeth. Pop some gum in your mouth. If you can get your mind off the craving for just a while, it will often go away.

You can also try taking preemptive strikes. If you find yourself regularly craving sweets at 10 p.m., shift one of your daily snacks from mid-afternoon to 8:30 p.m. If need be, have one of your allowable dark chocolate bites at that time. Savour the taste and make it last longer than the later craving pleaser ever would. It's better to indulge slowly in a small square of dark bittersweet chocolate at 8:30 than devour a candy bar at 10.

WHEN THE SCALE WON'T BUDGE

Just as every dieter fights cravings, every dieter gets stuck on plateaus from time to time as well. Our bodies don't always behave the way we want them to. So even though we're following the diet guidelines to a T (or believe we

---

EATING: The Sonoma Diet Way
Another good temporary measure for stopping excessive snacking is to meet your cravings halfway. Treat yourself to a smaller, healthier version of the food you're craving. If you think you need a bag of potato crisps, slice a quarter of a sweet potato instead. Brush the slices with a little olive oil and sprinkle salt or an herb over them. Bake the slices in an oven at 190°C/375°F/gas mark 5 until they're crisp. Satisfaction guaranteed, without the unhealthy carbs and fats, and many fewer calories.

are), we sometimes hit periods when the scale needle simply refuses to move. It doesn't seem fair, but it happens.

Your first and best reaction is to wait it out. Stick to your good eating habits and don't let yourself get frustrated. It's usually a matter of days before you start dropping the pounds again.

Plateaus are often easily explainable. The most likely plateau period is the shift from Wave 1 to Wave 2. Remember, you're actually adding calories to your diet at this point, as well as a number of new foods. Water retention, an adjustment in blood sugar metabolism, and other factors could conspire against weight loss as you settle into Wave 2. Ride it out.

But if the plateau drags on for a week, or you're actually gaining weight, it's time to take a look at what's going on. Adjustments are in order.

The first thing you need to do is make sure you're following the diet guidelines correctly. It's not uncommon for a dieter to be firmly convinced that he or she is adhering faithfully to the rules, only to discover upon closer examination that something's out of kilter.

Again, this is where a food journal can help you get to the bottom of things. But whether you keep a journal or not, take a close inventory of your eating habits to see where you may be going wrong.

Are you following the plate proportions fairly closely? Are you heaping the portions into something resembling the Egyptian pyramids? Are you using a plate that's the wrong size?

Are you pulling fruits and vegetables off the wrong tier lists? Has your snacking got out of hand? (Remember, a Tier 1 vegetable is the best snack unless you really need something more.) Are you choosing cuts of red meat that aren't as lean as they should be?

Are your breads and cereals 100% whole grain or are refined grains also included? (Check the labels with an eagle eye.) Are you cheating on the sweets? Are extra fat portions sneaking into your meals or snacks?

Go through your entire eating regimen with a fine-tooth comb. Pledge anew to be a real stickler to the rules, at least until your weight starts dropping again. Chances are you'll see some movement soon. The Sonoma Diet will always work—but only if you follow it.

Back on Track

If you hit a plateau where you stop losing weight, it will almost always happen on Wave 2. One option you can consider is going back through Wave 1 again. This is probably your best bet if your self-inspection confirms that you're indeed meeting the diet guidelines. In that case, another 10 days of Wave 1 will surely get you back on track for the simple reason that fewer calories are built into the meal plans.

You should also consider going back through Wave 1 if you suspect that your failure to continue losing weight has something to do with sugar cravings or white bread cravings. You know best, of course, whether you've been eating sugared sweets or any kinds of grains that aren't whole. Either of these transgressions on a regular basis will stop your weight loss every time.

If that's the case, a rerun of Wave 1 is called for because you still need to kick your addiction to sugar and refined white flour. Your blood sugar metabolism hasn't adjusted to a better diet yet. Your body simply isn't ready for the higher calorie consumption of Wave 2.

If that's the case, another 10 days of Wave 1 should do the trick. Not only will you be eating fewer calories, you'll also consume close to zero sugar—not even fruits. You'll need to redouble your efforts to stay sugar-free and refined flour-free for those 10 days. That means no bread, crackers, or pasta of any kind that isn't whole grain—and even less of the whole grain versions than on Wave 2.

You absolutely must get sugar and white flour out of your system before you can reap the full benefits of Wave 2.

Get Moving

A high priority for keeping your weight loss going at full clip is to increase your physical activity. Some kind of exercise that you enjoy is vital for efficient weight loss and optimum health.

On the Sonoma Diet, you should do some exercise from the very beginning of Wave 1. The main reason for this requirement is simple. The Sonoma Diet is not a low-carbohydrate diet. You're eating grains and lots of vegetables from the get-go, plus the carbs in your dairy. The first and best use of a consumed carbohydrate is to be burned as energy. The second and worst use is to be stored as fat.

More physical activity means more energy use. More energy use means more carbohydrate and body fat is burned and therefore less is stored as body fat. That may be a rather simple way of putting it, but it's basically why exercise helps you lose weight.

Calories are nothing but energy units. Burn as many calories as you consume, and your weight stays put. Burn more than you consume, and you lose weight. The Sonoma Diet takes care of providing just enough calories for you to be able to lose weight without feeling unsatisfied. Your contribution will be to burn more of those calories through exercise to lose weight even quicker.

And of course you'll gain the health benefits of exercise itself. Those benefits are so well documented and so widely disseminated that we won't bother you with a rehash here. Suffice it to say that the heart-protective effect of regular cardiovascular exercise—that is, endurance activity such as walking, running, biking, stair climbing, or swimming—fits in perfectly with the healthy approach of the Sonoma Diet. Much of the longevity and low incidence of heart disease amongst the peoples of the Mediterranean is attributed to their active lifestyles as well as their healthy diet.

SO WHAT DO I DO FOR EXERCISE?

This is a diet book. It's already plenty long with the diet instructions, diet advice, meal plans, and recipes. So we're going to spare you a lot of exercise instruction. There's plenty of that to be found elsewhere.

We're not going to badger you about exercising, either. The Sonoma Diet will get you to your target weight with or without exercise. You will get there faster, however, if you do some exercise, even a little bit. You will also be healthier and feel better if you exercise.

Those are the facts. Whether you exercise or not (and how much) is up to you. We trust you to make the best decision for your situation.

There are some factors to keep in mind, however, especially if you've never done five minutes of exercise in your life. First and most important, find a form of physical activity that you enjoy. Do what you like, rather than what somebody else tells you is "the best." If exercise is drudgery for you, or something you dread, you're not going to stick with it.

The second piece of essential advice is to start off easy. At the beginning, what or how much you do matters a lot less than simply doing something regularly. Just take a walk around the block after lunch or dinner. Play tag with your kids. Shoot some baskets. The important thing is to get in the habit of doing something physical every day. Then you can gradually work your way up to the half hour of sustained activity recommended for improving cardio-vascular health.

BENEFITS OF EXERCISE

Increases Energy Level

Improves Sleep Patterns

Enhances the Immune System

Decreases Arthritis

Protects Against Some Cancers

Decreases Heart Disease Risk Factors

Wards Off Depression

Accelerates and Maintains Weight Loss

Reduces Muscular Tension

Improves Bone Health

Decreases Stress Levels

Strength training—that is, any kind of activity that makes your muscles work more than they're used to—also has weight-loss benefits. That's because firmer, better-toned muscles increase what's known as your lean body mass, which is basically everything that's not body fat. The research shows that the higher your percentage of lean body mass, the more efficient your metabolism operates. That means quicker weight loss.

This kind of strength-increasing exercise (such as jogging, biking, and swimming) complements your cardio training. You can start out with a simple pair of light dumbbells to work with at home or join a gym and take advantage of the full range of weights and machines built for easy use. Even regular gardening will help tone your muscles, as anyone who's ever weeded or dug soil will testify.

The main thing is to approach exercise as something fun. You may feel a little awkward at first, no matter what you do. But if you smile your way through it and be persistent, your body will let you know how much it appreciates the chance to move. You'll feel better and lose weight faster.

WAVE 3:
THE SONOMA
DIET LIFESTYLE

Wave 3 of the Sonoma Diet starts the day you reach your target weight.

Okay, let's put that a little more realistically. Wave 3 starts the day after you reach your target weight. Because when the scale finally reads out that magic number you've been shooting for, you'll probably feel more like celebrating than thinking about the next wave.

That's perfectly understandable. So go ahead and celebrate. You've earned it.

The fact is, you've accomplished much more than a healthy, happy (and great-looking) body weight. By following through on Waves 1 and 2 of the Sonoma Diet, you've changed your entire approach to eating—for the better.

You've rid your body and mind of their fattening dependence on white bread, rolls, crackers, and other bakery foods made from refined flour. You've replaced them with satisfying amounts of fibre-laden and richer-tasting whole grain breads and cereals.

You've eliminated sugar cravings so that sugar-sweetened items are back to being what they're meant to be—occasional treats. By breaking yourself of the sugar habit, you've rediscovered that the wholesome natural sweetness of fresh ripe fruits and berries makes for as rewarding a dessert experience as you could ever want.

You've banned harmful hydrogenated fats from your diet and learned to keep saturated fats down to the bare miminum. At the same time, you haven't succumbed to an irrational fear of fat; instead you've taken advantage of reasonable amounts of the healthy and weight-friendly dietary fats in olive oil, nuts, avocados, and fish.

Most important, you've made the three-way connection between eating for pleasure, eating for health, and eating to stay at your best weight. You no longer see life as a choice between enjoying food and staying slim. On the contrary, you've discovered for yourself that the most efficient way to reach your ideal body weight is to revel in the pleasure that the healthiest and most naturally delicious foods have to offer.

You didn't just learn these lessons. You put them into practice. It wasn't always easy, especially at first. But by now you should have the results to show for your efforts—an ideal weight, the slimmer body you've always wanted, a healthier heart, clothes that fit right, oodles more energy, a boosted sense of self-esteem, and a heartfelt appreciation of the almost spiritual joy that can be experienced by slowly savouring a delicious, healthy meal with family or friends.

In short, you're living the Sonoma Diet lifestyle.

REAP THE REWARDS

Wave 3 is all about extending that lifestyle from a weight-loss strategy to a permanent way of existing happily on this planet. It comes down to enjoying food and all the other good things life has to offer without worrying about being overweight. Wave 3 is the time for you to reap the rewards of the Sonoma Diet lifestyle.

Live it to the hilt. Keep finding new sources of variety for your meals. Foods from all over the world are finding their way into every nook

What people are saying about Sonoma ...

"The Sonoma Diet has helped me return to the basics— eating healthy, making healthy choices, and increasing my physical activity. It isn't so much a diet as it is a lifestyle." Eva, age 57, weight loss to date: 22 lb

and cranny. Try whatever you can find, as long as it meets the Sonoma Diet guidelines.

All kinds of exotic and delicious fruits and vegetables are becoming available, many that you won't find on our lists. On Wave 3, you're free to experiment with them.

Keep pushing that health and pleasure connection. Now that weight loss is no longer the main factor in your meal planning, the satisfaction you'll get from enjoying reasonable portions of healthy, wholesome foods is actually increased. You're eating well for its own sake. And that feels great.

YOUR PERFECT WEIGHT FOR LIFE

Your first order of business for Wave 3, of course, is to stay at your ideal weight. This is what's often called "maintenance" in diet circles. But that's not the word of choice here.

There's nothing technically wrong with the term—you are, after all, seeking to "maintain" a certain weight. But "maintenance" sounds like something for aeroplane engines, not human beings. What you really want to do in Wave 3 is enhance the benefits of the Sonoma Diet lifestyle. Do that, and your weight maintenance will take care of itself.

For example, you've made the effort to turn at least one of your daily meals into a long and leisurely affair in which you eat slowly and savour every bite. You know that this elementary step not only turns mealtime into a soul-satisfying, sociable experience, it also works wonders for weight control by helping you eat less and digest better.

On Wave 3, you can work on turning the other two meals into similar experiences. True, for most of us lunchtime isn't as conducive to a leisurely pace as dinner. But chances are it can be considerably more leisurely than what you've been accustomed to.

Same for breakfast. Yes, you're rushed. Everybody's rushed in the morning. But do you really have to be rushed to the point of semi-panic? Connoisseurs of the Sonoma Diet lifestyle will wake up a half hour earlier each morning and use

SHOPPING: The Sonoma Diet Way

Visit farmers' markets when they're in season. Local farmers are often the first to introduce new varieties to an area, and they usually provide the freshest and most interesting produce.

the time to slow down at breakfast. Enjoy your coffee or tea. Take it easy. Every extra second you take during any meal makes it that much easier to keep your weight down.

Another way to intensify your Sonoma Diet lifestyle is by seeking more ways to have fun through physical activity. By Wave 3, whatever exercise plan you've chosen should have become a habit—that is, it's by now such a routine part of your day that you feel uncomfortable any time you miss a walk, a jog, or whatever workout you had scheduled.

EATING: The Sonoma Diet Way

If you must have lunch at your desk, at least turn off the computer and stay off the phone while you're eating. Better yet, take it somewhere else—the lunchroom, a park bench, anywhere you can dedicate yourself to enjoying your meal rather than putting food in your mouth while doing something else.

You'll of course continue to do your regular exercise. Your heart and your weight won't have it any other way. But for Wave 3, you'll want to look for opportunities to challenge yourself physically, doing things that have nothing to do with exercise as a routine. In Sonoma County, for example, biking and hiking are as normal for most people as breathing and sleeping are for people elsewhere.

Wherever you live, get used to taking a walk after dinner instead of flipping on the television. Or go bowling or hiking instead of to the movies on a weekend. Just for the heck of it, take the stairs instead of the escalator or lift. Spend some time pottering in the garden on a regular basis.

These are little things, to be sure, but they help keep the weight off and your energy up. And, conveniently, having the weight off makes these little activities more appealing. They also accumulate to create an active lifestyle. Your life will be richer, healthier, and a lot more fun.

It's Your Own Diet Now

Your actual diet instructions for Wave 3 come down to one rule: Do whatever you think is best for staying within the guidelines of the Sonoma Diet. Now that may sound impossibly open-ended, but it's based on a simple fact. You know by now what works best for you. So continue to do it.

You know, for example, that white bread and other refined flour products are an open invitation to weight gain and metabolic problems. You will continue to stay away from them almost all the time. Sweets are no longer part of your life; they are special treats and nothing more. In addition, you realize that saturated and hydrogenated fats are just as unhealthy for people at their best weight as they are for overweight people. Don't eat them.

The "basic guidelines" also include the plate proportions you became used to in Wave 2. For lunch and dinner, that means equal parts grains, fruit, vegetables, and either protein or dairy. You're used to reasonable portion sizes now as well, and you should stick with them—though you can estimate the amounts instead of using the same 18- and 23-cm/7- and 9-inch plates. (You may have already switched to estimates long ago; that's fine as long as you're hitting the sizes and proportions close to the real thing.)

You'll also want to keep your kitchen stocked with the Sonoma Diet foods. There's no need to keep unhealthy foods in your cabinets. And chances are you don't want to see them there anyway.

The food lists you've been using are still operative and always will be. Continue to eat more of the Tier 1 vegetables and the Tier 2 fruits and vegetables than those on Tier 3. Continue to avoid the foods you've been avoiding since Day 1—fatty meats, fruit juices, potatoes, full-fat dairy products, hydrogenated fats, refined grains, and sugared sweets.

These are guidelines you've been following from the start. Again, they're lifestyle choices. The only difference now is that you're following them for health and weight maintenance reasons, and no longer for weight loss. They're just as important as ever.

Your Beautiful Reward

The reason Wave 3 is easier on the Sonoma Diet than equivalent "maintenance" phases on other diets is that the eating plan for the bulk of the diet (Wave 2) was essentially designed to be sustainable for life. The typical Sonoma dieter enjoys meals more during Wave 2 of the diet than she or he did before the diet started. So there's no eagerness to get back to the old ways once the weight goal is reached. If you've ever been on a diet before, you know what it's like to sit at a table and have to graciously assure everyone else at the table that you are fine eating a different meal from what the others are enjoying. Well, the truth is, that's miserable for you and everyone else. The Sonoma Diet is centred on foods that can be enjoyed by everyone. You need only fill your plate according to the Sonoma Diet plate diagrams—with the same delicious foods everyone at the table will be enjoying.

With low-carb or low-fat diets, on the other hand, you achieve your weight loss by sticking to an eating plan based on artifically reduced amounts of needed foods. So naturally you and your body are ready and willing to make up for lost nutrition, so to speak, and overeat carbs or fat to compensate. That's where the infamous yo-yo effect or "rebounding" comes in.

With the Sonoma Diet, that's less of an issue because you've been eating satisfying and well-balanced meals the whole time. You haven't been "depriving" yourself of white bread and sweets, waiting for the day you can have them again. Rather, you've kicked the white bread and sweets habit and replaced them with better alternatives. That's not a sacrifice. That's a positive change for life.

Still, you do have more slack on Wave 3 of the Sonoma Diet. There are indeed some little extras you can afford yourself without compromising the basic guidelines of the diet.

That makes perfect sense when you think about it. The rules so far, strictly interpreted, were designed to get you to steadily lose weight. Well, you've lost the weight by Wave 3 and you don't need to lose any more. If you continue to eat exactly as you did on Wave 2, you'll keep losing weight. You don't want that. You want to stay where you are. That means you can implement some subtle changes.

But it does not mean you can start eating refined flour products again, or sweets, or fatty meats, or any of the other no-nos you've eliminated. It does not mean you can ignore the proportions you've been following or the portion sizes. To repeat, the guidelines hold. All you want to do is tweak them in healthy ways.

What people are saying about Sonoma ...
"I am so excited about this diet and my [weight loss] success that I feel like I'm about to explode! Of all the diets I have tried, this one is an easy transition for a lifestyle change. Because it uses everyday-type foods loaded with flavour from herbs and spices, I look forward to each and every meal."
Marv, age 42, weight loss to date: 40 lb

Healthy Adjustments

By far the most recommended tweak is to boost your servings of fruits and vegetables. This obeys the most basic bylaw of the Sonoma Diet lifestyle— get the maximum amount of nutrients for the minimum number of calories. More fruits and vegetables will be even better for your heart and overall health. You'll probably find you can add several servings per day and stay at your best weight. Try this strategy first.

Another surprisingly effective weight maintenance technique is to allow yourself a forbidden treat once in a while. Don't force down a doughnut you don't really want. But now you can be a good sport and try the birthday cake at a friend's party you otherwise would have declined. You can indulge in that sinful-looking pastry on the dessert trolley at a fancy restaurant you only visit on special occasions. You can even have pancakes and syrup (usually a white flour and sugar atrocity) on a special Sunday.

In other words, you don't have to be better than the rest of the world 365/24/7. Just something close to that.

You can get away with these treats now for three reasons. One is that you've worked hard and you deserve it. And unlike before, you're not doing it out of habit, but choice. You feel that it's a special indulgence, not a desperate need. That's okay.

Special Indulgences

Now that you've reached your target weight, you should be able to indulge in a treat for special occasions. Don't let yourself slide into eating a treat every day, or even every week. Make sure when you do indulge, you select a delectable treat that's really worth it to you—not just some stale brownies left in the lunchroom. Some special treats you may choose to indulge in include:

Butter
Dark Chocolate
Desserts, Pastries
Juices, Smoothies, or Energy Drinks
Potatoes
Pretzels, Crisps
Regular Fizzy Drinks

But most important, you can do it because your metabolism has actually changed for the better. This is one of the most vital and overlooked elements of weight loss. It's also one of the great advantages of being on Wave 3 after shedding pounds the healthy way on the Sonoma Diet. Let's take a look at what it means.

It may have occurred to you that for all their healthy dietary habits, many French and Italians and other Mediterraneans eat their share of white bread, pasta, and sweets. How do they get away with it? Well, some don't, of course. There's such a thing as an overweight Mediterranean or an overweight individual in Sonoma.

But most do get away with it because they eat that stuff in small amounts, and it's offset by a lifetime of olive oil, fruits, vegetables, wine, whole grains, and other dietary pluses that mark the Mediterranean diet. And they don't carry a spare tyre around their waists, so their metabolism is able to deal with the sugar and refined flour.

Your situation was probably quite the opposite when you first picked up this book. You were overweight, and you ate sweets and refined flour products habitually. Overweight people have more problems with insulin release and blood sugar control after eating sweets and refined flour, which is a big reason why they are overweight.

So you were spinning in a vicious cycle. That's why, you'll recall, the sugar and white flour prohibition was so strict from Day 1 of the diet. You simply had to get off that merry-go-round.

And at Wave 3 you are indeed off it. And you're no longer overweight. So your metabolism is in much better condition to deal with blood sugar rushes brought on by occasional forays into white bread and sugar territory. As long as they're occasional, you can handle it.

IF THINGS GO WRONG

What happens if your weight starts to creep up again? First of all, understand that there's no shame in this, and it's certainly nothing to panic about. In fact, it's likely to happen to even the most dedicated devotees of the Sonoma Diet lifestyle at some point in their lives. Things can happen. And this is exactly why Wave 3 exists. It's a built-in safety net.

The most obvious reason for the new weight gain is that you've over-tweaked. In other words, your adjustment from weight loss to maintenance went a little too far, and it's showing on the scale.

You may have added too much in the way of extra fruits or breads, or let your portions edge up a little bit extra, or overdone it with the "occasional" treats. Take it back a notch. Go easier on the extra fruits and breads, watch your portions, and add some extra days between those treats. Make sure you're not oversnacking too.

It's possible that re-tweaking won't get your weight back down fast enough for your satisfaction. That's okay too. The solution is to simply go back on Wave 2 until you've re-hit your ideal weight. You're an old hand at this after all, so it's simply a question of sticking to the Wave 2 guidelines again. That's what they're there for, and you may be reverting to them more than once over the years. Good health is a lifetime commitment.

The most drastic action you'll have to take on Wave 3 comes only if you find yourself not just regaining weight but slipping into the old sugar and white flour habits. And even this action isn't all that drastic. But you do have to nip this relapse in the bud, and the way to do that is to revert not to Wave 2 but all the way back to Wave 1.

Remember that Wave 1 is characterized by a total ban on sweet foods, even sugarless desserts. Fruits, with their natural sugars, are also on hold. Stick to all the guidelines of Wave 1, including limiting yourself to Tier 1 vegetables and using the Wave 1 plate percentages.

After 10 days, move to Wave 3 if you're back at your target weight. If not, go on to Wave 2 and stay there until your weight is where it needs to be.

DIET SURVIVAL 101

It's 10 p.m., you're all alone, and you're suddenly threatened by a vicious urge to devour a plate of nachos. What do you do? Whom do you call?

Diet emergencies can strike even the most dedicated Sonoma dieter. That's why we've included this chapter—to provide you with quick solutions to urgent problems when you need them the most.

Consider these pages your diet hotline, the place to go during a diet crisis. The emphasis here is on quick answers. You find more detailed strategies in "Fast-Track Your Weight Loss" beginning on page 94.

We'll start with solutions for the direst of emergencies. Then we'll run down strategies for dealing with less urgent problems.

EMERGENCY SERVICE

I'm absolutely craving sugar on Wave 1, and you won't even let me have artificial sweeteners. Mercy, please!

It's true that even artificial sweeteners are discouraged in Wave 1 to help you overcome your lifelong sugar addiction. Be strong, and you'll find you can do without sugary sweets by the end of Wave 1. And it's definitely worth it, because you can't eat sugar and lose weight at the same time. Plus, the natural goodness of fruits and vegetables comes out more when you're cured of the sugar habit.

Just when you think you are ready to give in, go one more day before you call it an emergency situation. That one day often makes the difference! Then if you really can't make it 10 days without something sweet, allow yourself some sugar-free gelatine or an artificial sweetener in your tea or coffee. That's a lot better than breaking down and eating an entire cheesecake! But it's still a stopgap. Try to have a sweetless day the day after each of these indulgences.

If you can just hang on 10 days until Wave 2, you'll have several non-sugar sweet options. Ideally, you'll want them less by that time, but they'll be available.

Help! I've stopped losing weight completely on Wave 2.
Make sure you're following the guidelines faithfully. Here's a checklist:

____ My plates and bowls are the right size.
____ I'm filling the plate with the right percentages of grains, protein, fruits, vegetables, and dairy.
____ I'm not heaping the portions.
____ I'm not surpassing my three daily fat servings.
____ The red meat I'm choosing is very lean.
____ I'm not eating the dark meat of poultry, and I'm getting rid of the chicken skin.
____ I'm not eating extra servings of Tier 2 or 3 vegetables.
____ I'm snacking just enough to satisfy between-meal hunger.
____ The breads and cereals I'm eating are truly 100% whole grain.
____ No sugar is sneaking into my diet.

I still can't get used to doing without white bread and a sugared dessert. So naturally I'm not losing weight any more now that I'm on Wave 2. Any suggestions?
You need to go through Wave 1 again. That will solve both your problems. You'll start losing weight again, because the calorie count is lower on Wave 1. Also, you need 10 more days of no sweet foods—not even sugarless desserts and fruits—to kick your sugar and white flour habit. Once you do, Wave 2

will be more enjoyable and more efficient. You'll lose weight without craving sweet things and white flour.

My weight loss is going way too slow. I'll never have the patience to keep it up at this rate.
Your best bet is to take up exercise if you haven't already done so. Even a minimum amount of physical activity—walking a half hour a day, for example, will help you burn off calories.

Also, choose vegetables only from Tier 1 and fruits only from Tier 2. Don't fill your plate to the edges; just that slight decrease in portion size will pay off as days go by (and you'll still be eating more calories than on Wave 1). Choose skinless chicken and fish more often than red meat as your protein serving. Eat even slower; you'll eat less that way.

I still crave some foods like crazy. Sometimes I'll give in and down a ton of salty snacks like potato crisps or devour enough chocolate bars for a week. Stop me before I strike again!
As soon as you feel a craving coming on, go do something else that doesn't involve food. Go for a walk. Take a shower. Call a friend on the phone—and not a mobile or portable you can carry into the kitchen with you. Cravings are often temporary. Stall them.

Or put something else in your mouth, such as gum or a sugar-free drop.

Distract yourself from the craving by eating something acceptable—a Tier 1 vegetable or some other allowable snack.

Drink a huge glass of water. Or a sugar-free fizzy drink. Sometimes what's triggering your craving is really thirst.

Eat a "lite" version of the food you're craving. A square of dark, bittersweet chocolate is an allowed occasional sweet. Have one if a chocolate craving hits but distance yourself from the rest of your chocolate stash. Instead of giving into potato crisp cravings, bake some salted slices of a sweet potato, sprayed with a little olive oil.

ADVICE AND CONSENT
Now that we've got the major crises taken care of, what about all the other nagging questions that come to you as you work your way through the diet?

Every Sonoma dieter experiences doubts or confusion. In fact, we've seen that it's mostly the same topics that pop up from time to time.

So here's the Sonoma Diet version of FAQs—frequently asked questions—with the answers that will help you get the most out of your diet. They're given here in no particular order. Let's just fire away.

What if I eat out a lot?

Simply order according to the food guidelines and eat controlled amounts that correspond to the plate percentages (usually 25% each of protein, whole grain, fruit, and vegetables). Rare is the restaurant that doesn't offer options that fit into the Sonoma Diet.

Even fast food places have salads with low-calorie dressings, grilled chicken breasts, lean turkey, or vegetable broth-based soups. At regular restaurants, it's easy to order a chicken or fish dish or a lean cut of red meat. Fruits and vegetables are always there for the asking. Just don't be a slave to the way things are presented on the menu; order exactly what you want.

Someone to Lean On

There's nothing like a comrade in arms to help you get the most out of a diet and smooth over the rough spots. If a friend or family member joins you on the Sonoma Diet, you're both way ahead of the game. You'll have somebody to call when cravings hit, somebody to talk to when things get hard, and somebody to share your experiences with.

You will have to make a few special requests. Wave away the bread basket, hold the butter or creamy sauces, and skip any cheese, croutons, or the like. Get your entree without white rice or potato; if they offer brown rice, that's great. If not, there's always that whole wheat roll for your whole grain. Many restaurants are great about making individual salads that contain lean cuts of protein with a vinaigrette. Take some ideas from the Sonoma Diet salads; they are made with ingredients that most restaurants stock. Describe a specific Sonoma Diet salad and see if they will prepare it.

Most waiters are used to special requests, and any restaurant worth eating at will gladly accommodate you. Always remember that you're there to eat what you want and enjoy yourself. You'll be surprised at how easy and fun it is to eat out and still stick to the Sonoma Diet guidelines.

How do I deal with food pushers like Aunt Agnes at family gatherings?

If the family gathering is once a year at Thanksgiving, go ahead and accept what she insists on serving—but eat very slowly and talk a lot. You can keep the damage to a minimum and make Aunt Agnes happy at the same time.

If the family meals are more frequent, take the offensive. Briefly explain that you're trying a new style of eating and that some foods just don't fit into your new eating plan. Ask her to help by not insisting you eat what you'd prefer to avoid. Then no matter what she says or does, eat what you'd planned on eating and no more. She'll get the picture . . . eventually.

What if I don't want wine or can't have it?

Simple. Don't drink it. Wine is voluntary.

What do I do with recipes that have different food types in them—such as a grain and vegetable medley? How do I apply that to the percentages?

You can tell from the ingredients in the recipe how much of each food type is in there. Then adjust accordingly. For example, if a dish consists of equal parts whole grains, protein, and vegetables, your task is easy. Simply spoon it out to fill three quarters of your plate and add a fruit to fill the last quarter. You now have the 25-25-25-25 ratio that most Wave 2 meals call for.

If the recipe dish is, say, mostly protein with some vegetables, consider it a protein dish. Use it to fill a tad more than the 25% of the plate reserved for protein and make up the missing vegetables with another vegetable.

As you can see, this is not a precise science. But you can come pretty close to the right percentages by using a little bit of estimating, some basic maths, and a good dose of common sense. And it gets easier as you progress into the diet and get used to the plate and the percentages.

Will this diet affect any medications I'm on?

Possibly. But most any change in lifestyle—including changes in eating, exercise, and weight—can. Or the medications may affect the diet. That's one reason why you must see your doctor before starting the Sonoma Diet.

All I want when I wake up in the morning is a steaming mug of coffee loaded with cream and sugar. Is this a no-no?
Yes and no. If you can't stand the thought of rolling out of bed unless there's a trip to the coffeepot in the near future, don't despair. You can drink two cups of black coffee per day—then switch to tea. When it comes to sugar, however, you're out of luck. Although artificial sweeteners are okay in small amounts, sugar is not. Try some of the premium coffees on the market now; you may find them good enough not to need your cream. If you absolutely cannot drink black coffee, you can add up to one tablespoon of heavy cream to your drink as long as you limit yourself to one mug per day instead of two. More involved coffee drinks, such as mochas, are to be avoided. They contain too many calories with little to no nutrients to show for them.

I hate green tea. What other tea can I drink?
Green tea's the best because it has high levels of antioxidants. Plus, some studies have shown that it boosts your metabolism, helping you burn more calories. White tea is great, too, but is more expensive and harder to find. If you really can't stomach it, however, black tea is an acceptable alternative. Most herbal teas (which usually have no caffeine) are okay as well.

I like the idea of a glass of wine at a meal, but I'm confused by it. How do I know what wines are appropriate and what goes with what?
Forget about all that. On the first day, decide how much money you can spend on a bottle of wine and buy one with a name you like. If you enjoy the wine, buy it again. If you don't, try another one. Or try one a friend recommends. The only wine rule that matters is to drink what you like and don't drink what you don't like. The way to find out what you like is to try different wines.

This diet is too expensive with all the protein, fruits, and vegetables. Is there a cheaper version?
The Sonoma Diet can push your grocery bill up a bit with its emphasis on fresh, wholesome foods. But there are tricks for keeping the cost down.

You can stock up on frozen and canned fruits and vegetables (as long as they have no added sugar). Some fresh vegetables are cheaper than others; if economy is a factor, let that decide which you buy. Fresh fruits and vegetables in season cost less. Some, such as berries, you can buy a lot of when the price is down and freeze them for later use. Check out farmers' markets; there are bargains, especially locally grown produce in season.

Look for what's on sale and make the diet work around that. For example, if chicken prices are way down this week (as they sometimes are), stock up and make chicken your protein for several days. Freeze the rest.

Look for bargains in bulk. That's often the case with beans and grains.

I'm one person and there's a whole bottle of wine ...

And since you should only drink one glass, what do you do with the rest? Actually, wine keeps longer than you think. You can buy rubber or plastic stoppers that fit tight with the help of a simple and inexpensive vacuum pump. Keep the stoppered white wine in the refrigerator and red wine in a

---

No Excuses

Are you an expert at finding reasons to fudge the diet guidelines? That puts you in the company of a large percentage of dieters. There's always a good excuse for eating a chocolate bar just this once, or for piling up the pork so it overflows the plate, or for going with white rice instead of brown. You're in a hurry, the pork would have been wasted, and the shop was out of brown rice. And so forth.

Excuses sabotage your diet. Deal with them. Get a piece of paper and a pen and write down all the excuses you use to eat what you shouldn't. Keep the paper and pen handy because you'll surely come up with new ones as the days go by.

Then alongside each excuse list a way to address it that makes sense for the way you live. If your excuse for eating a croissant in the morning instead of the prescribed Sonoma Diet breakfast is that you don't have time, write next to that excuse, "get up 15 minutes earlier." If your excuse for adding sugar to your coffee is "that's what I'm used to," write down "get used to artificial sweetener or unsweetened coffee."

True, writing down solutions is no guarantee you'll carry them out. But when you see in black and white how easy it can be to overcome your excuses, the solutions are harder to ignore. Try it.

---

spot that's not too warm. You should be able to drink it for at least two days, sometimes more.

I don't have the time to prepare my own meals. It takes too long.

Take shortcuts. Most of the actual work time is spent chopping and preparing. So buy pre-cut meats and vegetables when you can. For the rest, devote one hour at the beginning of the week to chop and prepare all the ingredients for a week's worth of meals. Then at mealtime it's just a question of putting them together and throwing them on the stove or in the oven.

Also, you can make, say, eight to 10 servings of grains at a time and just reheat the amount you will be eating for lunch or dinner each day for a week. Cook up lots of pinhead oatmeal at the beginning of the week and reheat it for breakfast every day. Or you can make scrambled eggs in about two minutes by mixing up a couple of eggs in a bowl, adding a little water, and microwaving it on high for a minute. Take it out and stir. Then microwave for another minute.

I don't have time to prepare the recipes.

You'll find you have more time than you thought once you realize how good and helpful the recipes are. Start by doing what you can and no more. Commit to preparing just two of the recipes in a week, even if it's just a side dish such as a grain or salad. Work your way up to four. Gradually, you'll be able to free up the time for preparing good meals. Remember, the recipes are there to give you variety so you aren't bored with your diet. They're also there to expose you to the Sonoma Diet way of cooking and the delicious possibilities of healthy food. That's worth making time for.

Others in my family insist on keeping non-Sonoma Diet food in the kitchen, so I'm surrounded by it.

The worst of that food—processed baked goods, biscuits, crackers, crisps, sugar-filled cereal—doesn't do anybody any good, whether on a diet or not. Lay down the law and banish it from the house. If it's not there, nobody will eat it—including you. And it's the least your family can do to support you.

Help them along. With the harmful food gone, put out fresh fruit in the kitchen. Have whole grain bread and peanut butter available. Stock up on vegetables and have some cut and ready for them to snack on. Let them see that a healthy kitchen is no deprivation.

I'm the only one in my family on the diet. That makes mealtime something of a struggle.
There's nothing odd about the food on the Sonoma Diet. Anyone can eat it and enjoy it. There's no reason why the meal you prepare for yourself can't be for everyone. Perhaps your family can eat a little more than you, but that should be the only difference.

Give them a challenge. Ask them to try the Sonoma Diet meals for a week. Serve your favourite recipes from the diet. See what happens. If they refuse to try the recipes, you can always serve them the meat dish that coincides with the Sonoma Diet recipe you're eating that night, and they can have their own side dishes. They can have it their way, you'll have it your way, and the conflict will at least be minimized. Anything that can be done to help all of you enjoy a slow meal together is beneficial for everybody.

I travel a lot and so my choices are often limited. Any suggestions?
Restaurant menus and the Sonoma Diet definitely can work together (see pages 129–131). And your choices on the road may not be as limited as you think. When staying out of town, seek out big supermarkets, health food shops, and even the farmers' market. They're as easy to find as any restaurant. And they always have available Sonoma Diet-style food. Some markets even offer fresh foods prepared and ready to eat.

I take my lunch to eat at work. What are my options?
There's not much on the Sonoma Diet that can't be prepared at home and brought to work for either microwaving or eating straight from the container. Specifically, bagged salad blends are good. Try different ones for variety. Top them with cooked chicken breasts, tuna, lean cold meats, or hard-boiled eggs. Add a fruit and a whole wheat roll and you have something pretty close to the usual lunch food proportions.

Other ideas: bring leftover lean steaks, chicken breasts, or fish to heat up at work. Look at the Sonoma Diet express recipes beginning on page 127 for easy-to-make wraps using a variety of ingredients. You can always bring frozen or canned fruits or vegetables to microwave or just open up. Cubed chicken, pork, or ham with a raw vegetable, an apple, and a whole grain roll or whole grain crackers gives you an easy and complete lunch. With a little creativity and some planning, you can pretty much have any lunch you want at work.

Do I have to exercise?

No. But you'll lose weight faster if you do. And you'll be healthier as you lose the weight. If you're really averse to the idea of exercise, start with something small and easy. Just walk. Keep track of how far you go and try to add a little each week. Even that small effort will help.

Where do I find the plates?

It's interesting how many people learn they don't have an 18-cm/7-inch or a 23-cm/9-inch plate in the house once they start the Sonoma Diet. If you don't want to buy a whole set of plates at the right size, you can always go to a secondhand shop, buy just enough unmatched, interesting plates for your family, and use them for the duration of the diet.

If that's out of the question, there's no rule against taking a bigger plate and only using 23 or 18 cm (9 or 7 inches) of it. If you have paper plates around, there's a good chance they're 23 cm/9 inches in diameter (check the package; it says somewhere on there). If they're the right size, you can either use the paper plates for the diet or put one over a bigger plate to see where the 23-cm/9-inch circle is. Then use that portion of the bigger plate.

I like to snack all day instead of eating three big meals. Can I spread my meals out throughout the day?

The Sonoma Diet is based on three meals a day—breakfast, lunch, and dinner. There are two reasons for this. One is that three squares is the way almost everybody eats. The other is that, at each meal, the three-a-day system gives you the beneficial food combinations we talked about earlier in the book.

If spreading out your meals is important to you, you can try it. You'll have to do the maths so that you're eating the same amount of food in the same percentages as you would on a three-a-day plan. But keep in mind that you'll be sacrificing the full benefit of the food combinations that are an important part of the Sonoma Diet.

I've got kids who are still mad at me for giving away all the ice cream and processed food when I started Wave 1. How do I keep them happy without tempting myself away from the diet?

The easy response would be to suggest storing their food in a separate cabinet and opening it only when feeding them. But there's a better answer.

Do your kids a favour and downplay those foods, reserving them for special treats. As a parent, your job is to buy healthy food and have it available for them. The children's job is to choose from what is offered. If what is offered is all healthy, the kids have to choose from only healthy food.

The best strategy is not to make a big deal out of the change. Wait for the crisp supply to run out, then don't refill it. Buy something Sonoma Diet-friendly to replace the crisps. Or when the biscuits run out, have packages of plain oatmeal around with a variety of toppings for a snack. They'll balk at first, but over time they'll get used to it and learn to love it.

What should I look for on food labels regarding carbs and sugar?

"Carbs" is too general a concept to deal with. Instead, choose baked goods and breads that contain whole grains as the primary ingredients. Avoid buying foods that contain sugar, especially as one of the first five ingredients. Sugar is often called many things, such as sucrose, fructose, dextrose, or high fructose corn syrup. A good rule is to look at fibre levels for whole grain breads. If there isn't any fibre, don't buy it. Generally, whole grain breads have at least 2 grams of fibre per slice, and cereals have 8 grams per serving.

Are canned and frozen vegetables okay?

Yes. Fresh is best, of course, but frozen is fine too. Canned is your third choice. Check the ingredient list to make sure sauces, sugar, or oils have not been added to the canned foods. Rinsing canned vegetables will cut down on the added salt.

How do I get enough protein if I don't want to eat eggs or meat?
If you eat fish, you're in fine shape. Fish is a great protein source with the added benefit of healthy omega-3 fats. If you don't want to eat fish either, you'll find other protein sources on the Sonoma Diet Proteins and Dairy list (page 75 for Wave 1; page 92 for Wave 2). They include beans and soya products.

Can I eat peanut butter?
Try all-natural peanut butter with no sugar or hydrogenated fats. Regular peanut butter has trans fats. Use the all-natural kind as an occasional snack in Wave 2. Dab a teaspoonful on a piece of whole grain bread or a fruit—the fats and protein in the peanut butter slow the blood sugar release of the carbohydrates in the bread or fruit.

Can I use butter?
In Wave 3, you can use butter as an occasional treat. Butter, whether it's in spray or stick form, is loaded with saturated fat. Margarine is not a substitute—it contains trans fats. Whenever possible, use olive oil.

What if I find a vegetable that's not on any list?
If it's starchy, such as a root vegetable, consider it Tier 3. If it's watery, such as a cucumber, it's probably low in calories and fibre rich. So you can treat it as a Tier 1 vegetable. In between the two? It's probably a Tier 2.

Can't I drink some kind of alcohol besides wine?
Not until you reach your target weight. Research has revealed some health benefits from alcohol in general, but only wine packs enough healthy nutrients to make the extra calories worth it. Also, among alcoholic beverages only wine contributes to the slow, leisurely, pleasurable aspect of a meal.

WELCOME TO THE MEAL PLANS AND RECIPES

The Sonoma Diet was designed to be two things above all else—simple and flavourful.

We promised you at the very beginning that we've done all the thinking and figuring for you. In this final section of the book, you'll reap the benefit. Here you'll find the recipes, meal plans, and food lists that will guide you through your weight-loss programme, one day at a time.

Flexibility is the key. You can follow the menu plans for each meal for the duration of the diet or you can use the information ahead to improvise your own meals within the diet's guidelines. It's your choice.

The bulk of this part of the book is recipes—dozens of them. They consist of easy-to-follow, step-by-step instructions for preparing mouthwatering dishes that will keep you satisfied as you shed pounds.

The recipes are nothing like what most people think of as "diet food." They feature international flavours inspired by Sonoma County's adventurous culinary style. Your taste buds will never be bored.

The recipes are divided into two sections. First come those that conform to the food choices for Wave 1 of your diet. Then you'll find the more varied Wave 2 recipes. You have the comfort of knowing that the recipe you choose will be 100% appropriate for your stage of the diet.

The sections on meal plans for Waves 1 and 2 offer daily menus to guide you through your diet. Simply by preparing and eating the suggested dishes for each meal of the day, you can progress through the Sonoma Diet on automatic pilot, with every meal planned out for you.

But if you want to improvise a bit— either to save time or add variety— you'll find plenty of suggestions for doing just that. For example, you always have the choice of substituting grilled or roasted chicken (skinless, of course) for any main dish. That gives you the time-saving option of preparing several days' worth of chicken breasts for the protein part of your plate. Use the Seasonings section to add flavour to your meal by choosing one of the rubs, marinades, or sauces for your chicken. If you're in the mood for a quick yet refreshing meal, create your own Sonoma Express Wrap or Sonoma Express Salad following the recipes on pages 127 and 128. And you'll maintain weight-loss success even when dining out if you follow the helpful advice on pages 129 through 131 for how to enjoy eating out without busting your diet.

SAVE TIME: Try Sonoma Express

When you need a quick lunch or dinner, make it easy on yourself by replacing any of the menu items in Wave 1 or 2 with a Sonoma Express Wrap, Sonoma Express Salad, or Sonoma Express Chicken (see recipes, pages 127 and 128). Be sure to choose Wave-appropriate vegetables based on where you are on the diet. If you're on Wave 2, be sure to include a serving of fruit with any of these meal substitutes.

SONOMA EXPRESS WRAP

These make quick and easy meal substitutes for when you're in a hurry or on the go. Fill your wrap with your choice of Sonoma-friendly ingredients or follow one of our recipe ideas (see pages 168, 172, 237, and 238). If you're on Wave 2, add a serving of fruit to your meal.

For one wrap

Use 1 low-carb, whole wheat tortilla, or a large lettuce leaf to wrap your ingredients.

Spread the tortilla or lettuce leaf with up to 1 tablespoon of your favourite spread.*

Fill it with:

85 g/3 oz mixed greens or spinach leaves

85 g/3 oz vegetables (be sure to choose Wave-appropriate vegetables based on where you are on the diet)

Cooked lean protein such as chicken, pork, beef, or ham. Use 85 g/3 oz for lunch or 115 g/4 oz for dinner.

50 g/2 oz (about 2 tablespoons) mozzarella cheese, low-fat cream cheese, or goat's cheese (optional)

*Note: See the Seasonings section (pages 133–159) for full-flavoured spreads such as Roasted Garlic Spread or Black Bean-Smoked Chilli Spread. If you're feeling pressed for time, use bought products such as roasted tomato salsa, artichoke spread, or hummus.

SONOMA EXPRESS SALAD

This salad is a simple way to use what you have on hand for lunch or dinner. If you're on Wave 2, add a serving of fruit to your meal.

For one salad

85 g/3 oz mixed greens or spinach leaves

85 g/3 oz vegetables (be sure to choose Wave-appropriate vegetables based on where you are on the diet)

115 g/4 oz cooked beans (canned work well) or have 2 crackers with your salad

Cooked lean protein such as chicken, pork, beef, ham, or eggs. Use 85 g/3 oz for lunch or 115 g/4 oz for dinner, or 2 eggs for either meal.

50 g/2 oz (about 2 tablespoons) mozzarella cheese, low-fat cream cheese, or goat's cheese (optional)

Choice of salad dressing*

*Note: See the Seasonings chapter (pages 133–159) for dressings such as Peppercorn-Strawberry Vinaigrette or Pesto Vinaigrette. Or use a bought low-calorie salad dressing.

SONOMA EXPRESS CHICKEN

For one serving

115 g/4 oz skinless, boneless chicken breast

Choice of rub or marinade from the Seasonings chapter (pages 133–159)

Grill or barbecue the chicken for about 15 minutes, turning once.

Note: The rub and marinade recipes make enough for 4 to 6 servings of meat, so it's easy to accommodate more servings. Cooking time remains the same.

EATING OUT

Enjoying meals at restaurants is a way of life in Sonoma County—and a true pleasure everywhere. The Sonoma Diet is designed so that you can eat out without missing a beat in your weight-loss programme.

But you do have to take action to stick with your Sonoma Diet meal plans and portion sizes when you're eating away from home. Your mission is to make sure that your restaurant meals are adjusted to your diet, not the other way around.

It's easier than you think. Most restaurants are happy to accommodate you. Even those places with more rigid menus—such as chains or fast food restaurants—have options that fit in with your meal plans.

Keep in mind the following strategies for taking the Sonoma Diet outside your home and you'll never have to put your diet on hold.

Tips for Dining Out

• **Phone ahead.** The surest way to know ahead of time if a restaurant will work with your food preferences is to ask them. Call during non-peak hours, explain very briefly what your general needs are, and see what they say.

• **Check out the menu online.** Many restaurants have a website, and often the menu is listed. If you can get an advance look at the menu, you can avoid any confusion or discomfort that might come from making a last-minute decision about what to request.

• **Engage the waiter.** Ask questions about how a dish is prepared if the menu is not clear. For example, is it cooked with animal fat or vegetable oil? How big is the portion? Any minimally competent server will be glad to answer or find out if he or she doesn't know.

• **Look for give-away words on the menu.** "Steamed," "in its own juice," "garden fresh," "grilled," "roasted," and "poached" usually indicate a lower-fat, lower-calorie preparation. The dish they describe is more likely to conform to the Sonoma Diet guidelines. On the other hand, consider the following words or phrases to be red flags: buttery, buttered, in butter sauce, fried, pan-fried, crispy, braised, creamed, in cream sauce, in its own gravy, hollandaise, au gratin, in cheese sauce, scalloped, marinated in oil, basted, casserole, hash, pot pie.

• **Seize control of your salad dressing.** Ask for extra-virgin olive oil and vinegar or reduced-fat or fat-free dressing. And order the salad dressing on the side so you can control how much you eat.

• **Have plenty of water.** Drink a glass before, during, and after your meal.

• **Watch your portion sizes.** Visualize the 450 ml/ $^3/_4$ pint bowl and the 18-cm/7-inch or 23-cm/9-inch plate as you're served. Arrange the food on the plate as you would at home to follow the prescribed proportions for the wave you're on. If decorum prevents you from doing this physically, do it in your mind. This gives you an idea of how much to eat.

• **Eat only the Sonoma Diet portion.** If you're served too much, put the excess in a takeaway box before you eat. Or share with your dining partner.

• **Order for two.** If you know in advance that the portions will be too large, consider splitting a meal with your dining partner.

• **Order what you want.** Don't be a slave to the menu. If it indicates that white rice comes with the salmon, ask for brown or wild rice instead. If that can't be done, ask them to substitute vegetables for the rice. Manipulate your order to approximate the grains/protein/vegetable/fruit proportions appropriate for the Sonoma Diet wave you're on.

• **Eat slowly.** Slow, pleasure-oriented dining is always a must on the Sonoma Diet. Enjoy your meal and the conversation that goes with it.

Restaurant Recommendations
Fast food burger chains

• Garden side salads with reduced-fat or fat-free salad dressing. Remove the crackers and cheese.

• Skinless, boneless chicken breast, grilled or chargrilled. Remove the bun. Eat it with a salad or use it to top your salad.

Fast food sandwich chains

• Low-carb, whole wheat tortilla filled with chicken or turkey breast, lean ham, or lean roast beef. Include spinach, tomato, pepper, onion, cucumber, or any other vegetables that are appropriate for your current diet wave.

• Add Dijon mustard or a reduced-fat or fat-free Italian salad dressing or a small amount of oil and vinegar for flavour.

• Add a tablespoon of Parmesan cheese or feta cheese.

Chinese restaurants
• Stir-fried skinless, boneless chicken breast, fish, prawns, scallops, lean beef, or lean pork. Ask them to leave the breading off the meat.
• Stir-fried vegetables, such as asparagus, broccoli, green beans, cabbage, cauliflower, courgettes, pak choi, and/or other appropriate vegetables.
• Stir-fried tofu, once you reach Wave 2. Make sure there's no breading.
• Only eat brown rice, and watch the portion size; estimate about 25 g/1 oz.

Italian restaurants
• Grilled skinless, boneless chicken breast, lean beef, lean pork, fish, prawns, lobster, scallops, mussels, and/or other shellfish flavoured with herbs and not breaded.
• Avoid creamy sauces.
• Ask for sautéed fresh vegetables tossed with a little extra-virgin olive oil.
• Avoid pasta unless whole wheat pasta is available. Watch the portion size.
• Choose a side salad with dark, leafy greens. Ask for fresh vegetables to top the salad. Drizzle a little extra-virgin olive oil and flavoured vinegar or reduced-fat or fat-free salad dressing over the salad.

Mexican restaurants
• Choose skinless, boneless chicken breast, lean beef, lean pork, prawns, or scallops.
• Choose black beans or whole bean soup instead of refried beans. Avoid the rice unless brown rice is available.
• Ask for a fresh guacamole or guacamole that is not prepared with added fat such as soured cream.
• Top meat with salsa, lettuce, and/or tomatoes; leave off the soured cream.

Buffets
• Sit as far away from the buffet table as possible.
• Fill your plate once, approximating the portion sizes and food-type proportions of the Sonoma Diet meal appropriate for your wave.
• Eat slowly—keep a little food on your plate until the last person at your

table is finished eating to avoid the temptation of accompanying your tablemates to the buffet for their second trip.

SEASONINGS

As you've read over and over throughout this book, the Sonoma Diet is all about full-flavoured, delicious food. This chapter offers you everything from rubs and marinades for meat and poultry to spreads for wraps to salad dressings you can use on salads, as marinades, or as dips and spreads. Don't be afraid to get creative with flavour!

And when you're in need of a quick and simple meal, try the following recipes for rubs, marinades, and spreads to enhance a Sonoma Express Wrap, Sonoma Express Salad, or Sonoma Express Chicken (see recipes, pages 127–128).

JAMAICAN JERK RUB

PREP: 5 MINUTES **CHILL:** 30 MINUTES
MAKES: ENOUGH FOR 450 g/1 lb MEAT OR POULTRY

70 g/2½ oz coarsely chopped onion
2 tablespoons lime juice
1 teaspoon crushed red pepper
½ teaspoon sea salt
¼ teaspoon ground allspice
¼ teaspoon curry powder
¼ teaspoon freshly ground black pepper
⅛ teaspoon dried thyme, crushed
⅛ teaspoon ground ginger
2 cloves garlic, quartered

1. In a blender combine onion, lime juice, crushed red pepper, sea salt, allspice, curry powder, black pepper, thyme, ginger, and garlic. Cover and blend until smooth. Sprinkle evenly onto 450 g/1 lb boneless pork chops, chicken breast halves, or turkey breast; rub in with your fingers. Cover and refrigerate for 30 minutes. Grill pork or poultry.

CHIPOTLE RUB

START TO FINISH: 5 MINUTES
MAKES: ENOUGH FOR 1.1 kg/2½ lb MEAT OR POULTRY

1 teaspoon ground coriander
¼ to ½ teaspoon freshly ground black pepper
¼ teaspoon paprika
1 small dried chipotle chilli, seeded and crushed,* or ⅛ to ¼ teaspoon cayenne pepper

1. In a small bowl stir together coriander, black pepper, paprika, and chilli. Sprinkle evenly onto 1.1 kg/2½ lb boneless pork chops, chicken breast halves, or turkey breast. Grill pork or poultry.

*Note: Because chillies contain oils that can burn your skin and eyes, wear rubber or plastic gloves when working with them. If your bare hands do touch the chillies, wash your hands well with soap and water.

FRESH HERB RUB

START TO FINISH: 5 MINUTES
MAKES: ENOUGH FOR 1.5 kg/3 lb MEAT, POULTRY, OR FISH

> 1 tablespoon chopped fresh thyme or ¾ teaspoon dried thyme, crushed
> 1 tablespoon chopped fresh sage or ¾ teaspoon dried sage, crushed
> 1 tablespoon chopped fresh rosemary or ¾ teaspoon dried rosemary, crushed
> 2 cloves garlic, minced
> 1½ teaspoons coarsely ground black pepper
> 1 to 1½ teaspoons sea salt
> ½ teaspoon crushed red pepper

1. In a small bowl stir together thyme, sage, rosemary, garlic, black pepper, sea salt, and crushed red pepper. Sprinkle evenly onto 1.5 kg/3 lb boneless pork chops, chicken breast halves, turkey breast, or fish fillets or steaks; rub in with your fingers. Grill pork, poultry, or fish.

MUSTARD-PEPPERCORN RUB

PREP: 5 MINUTES **CHILL:** 15 MINUTES TO 4 HOURS
MAKES: ENOUGH FOR 1.5 kg/3 lb MEAT

> 1 tablespoon coarse-grain mustard
> 2 teaspoons extra-virgin olive oil
> 2 teaspoons cracked black peppercorns
> 2 teaspoons chopped fresh tarragon or ½ teaspoon dried tarragon, crushed
> 1 teaspoon sea salt

1. In a small bowl stir together mustard, oil, peppercorns, tarragon, and sea salt. Spread evenly onto 1.5 kg/3 lb boneless beef steaks, boneless pork chops, or boneless lamb chops. Refrigerate for 15 minutes to 4 hours. Grill meat.

Asian Herb Marinade

PREP: 25 MINUTES **MARINATE:** 4 TO 24 HOURS
MAKES: ENOUGH FOR 900 g/2 lb PORK, CHICKEN, OR SALMON

6 tablespoons fresh coriander
50 g/2 oz cup minced fresh ginger
3 tablespoons fresh mint leaves
10 cloves garlic, halved
½ to 1 fresh serrano chilli, seeded and cut up*
1 tablespoon toasted sesame oil
1 tablespoon lime juice
1 teaspoon freshly ground black pepper
½ teaspoon sea salt

1. In a food processor combine coriander, ginger, mint, garlic, chilli, sesame oil, lime juice, black pepper, and sea salt. Cover and process to a thick paste, scraping down side of bowl as necessary.

2. To use as a marinade, spread over 900 g/2 lb pork tenderloin, chicken breast halves, or salmon steaks. Cover and chill in the refrigerator for 4 to 24 hours. Grill or roast pork or grill chicken or salmon.

*Note: Because chillies contain oils that can burn your skin and eyes, wear rubber or plastic gloves when working with them. If your bare hands do touch the chillies, wash your hands well with soap and water.

Tip: You can place the marinade in a freezer container; seal, label, and freeze for up to 3 months. Thaw before using.

Mediterranean Herb Marinade

PREP: 20 MINUTES **MARINATE:** 4 TO 24 HOURS
MAKES: ENOUGH FOR 900 g/2 lb PORK, CHICKEN, OR SALMON

6 tablespoons fresh flat-leaf parsley
50 ml/2 fl oz cup extra-virgin olive oil
3 tablespoons fresh rosemary leaves
3 tablespoons fresh thyme leaves
2 tablespoons coarsely chopped fresh sage
2 tablespoons finely shredded lemon peel
10 cloves garlic, halved
½ to 1 teaspoon crushed red pepper
½ teaspoon sea salt
¼ to ½ teaspoon freshly ground black pepper

1. In a food processor combine parsley, oil, rosemary, thyme, sage, lemon peel, garlic, crushed red pepper, sea salt, and black pepper. Cover and process to a thick paste, scraping down side of bowl as necessary.

2. To use as a marinade, spread over 900 g/2 lb pork tenderloin, chicken breast halves, or salmon steaks. Cover and chill for 4 to 24 hours. Grill or roast pork or grill chicken or salmon.

Tip: You can place the marinade in a freezer container; seal, label, and freeze for up to 3 months. Thaw before using.

CHERMOULA MARINADE

PREP: 10 MINUTES **MARINATE:** 8 TO 24 HOURS
MAKES: ENOUGH FOR 1.5 TO 1.8 KG/3 TO 4 lb FISH, POULTRY, BEEF, OR PORK

- 115 ml/4 fl oz extra-virgin olive oil
- 115 ml/4 fl oz lemon juice
  - 6 tablespoons chopped fresh flat-leaf parsley
  - 6 tablespoons chopped fresh coriander
  - 4 cloves garlic, minced
  - 1 tablespoon paprika
  - 2 teaspoons ground cumin
  - 1 teaspoon sea salt
  - ½ teaspoon cayenne pepper
  - ¼ teaspoon freshly ground black pepper

1. In a medium bowl whisk together oil, lemon juice, parsley, coriander, garlic, paprika, cumin, sea salt, cayenne pepper, and black pepper until combined.

2. To use as a marinade, place 1.5 to 1.8 kg/3 to 4 lb fish steaks, chicken breast halves, turkey breast, beef steaks, or boneless pork chops in a self-sealing plastic bag; pour lemon juice mixture over. Seal bag; turn bag to coat fish, poultry, or meat. Marinate in the refrigerator for 8 to 24 hours. Remove from marinade, discarding marinade. Grill fish, poultry, or meat. (Or serve as a sauce with grilled fish, poultry, or meat.)

TANDOORI MARINADE FOR CHICKEN

PREP: 15 MINUTES **MARINATE:** 4 HOURS
MAKES: ENOUGH FOR 450 TO 675 g/1 TO 1½ lb CHICKEN

  170 g/6 oz carton plain low-fat yogurt
  50 ml/2 fl oz lemon juice
  1 tablespoon grated fresh ginger
  2 tablespoons chopped fresh coriander
  2 cloves garlic, minced
  1 tablespoon cumin seeds, toasted and crushed*
  ½ teaspoon sea salt
  ¼ teaspoon cayenne pepper

1. In a small bowl stir together yogurt, lemon juice, ginger, coriander, garlic, cumin seeds, sea salt, and cayenne pepper.

2. To use as a marinade, place 450 to 675 g/1 to 1½ lb chicken breast halves in a self-sealing plastic bag; pour yogurt mixture over chicken. Seal bag; turn bag to coat chicken. Marinate in the refrigerator for 4 hours. Remove from marinade, discarding marinade. Grill chicken.

*Note: To toast seeds, heat a small frying-pan over medium heat. Add seeds. Cook about 2 minutes or until toasted and aromatic, shaking pan frequently. Place toasted seeds in a spice grinder and process until finely ground.

HONEY-MUSTARD MAYONNAISE

START TO FINISH: 10 MINUTES **MAKES:** ABOUT 170 ml/6 fl oz

  115 ml/4 fl oz light mayonnaise or salad dressing
  3 to 4 tablespoons honey mustard or coarse-grain Dijon-style mustard
  ⅛ teaspoon sea salt
  ⅛ teaspoon freshly ground black pepper

1. In a small bowl whisk together mayonnaise, mustard, sea salt, and black pepper. Use immediately or cover and chill for up to 1 week before using. Use as a spread for sandwiches and wraps.

Nutrition Facts per tablespoon: 45 cal., 4 g total fat (1 g sat. fat), 4 mg chol., 123 mg sodium, 2 g carbo., 0 g fibre, 0 g pro.

YOGURT AND CUCUMBER SAUCE

PREP: 30 MINUTES **CHILL:** 24 TO 48 HOURS **MAKES:** 450 g/1 lb

340 g/12 oz plain fat-free yogurt*
1 cucumber
¼ teaspoon sea salt
1 clove garlic, minced
½ teaspoon sea salt
1 tablespoon extra-virgin olive oil
1 tablespoon white wine vinegar
2 to 3 teaspoons dried mint, crushed, or 1 to 2 tablespoons chopped fresh mint
Fresh mint leaves (optional)
Toasted whole wheat pitta bread wedges, celery sticks, pepper strips, and/or broccoli or cauliflower florets (optional)

1. To make yogurt cheese, line a yogurt strainer, sieve, or a small colander with three layers of 100% cotton cheesecloth or a clean paper coffee filter. Suspend lined strainer, sieve, or colander over a bowl. Spoon yogurt into lined strainer, sieve, or colander. Cover with plastic wrap. Refrigerate for 24 to 48 hours. Discard liquid.

2. Cut the cucumber in half lengthwise. Remove the seeds. Slice the cucumber into 0.5-cm/¼-inch slices. Place slices in a bowl and toss with the ¼ teaspoon sea salt. Set aside for 15 to 30 minutes to draw out some of the liquid. Place cucumber in a colander. Rinse under cold water. Drain on paper towels.**

3. Meanwhile, using a mortar and pestle, mash garlic with the ½ teaspoon sea salt until a paste forms. In a large bowl combine oil, vinegar, and garlic paste. Stir in yogurt cheese and dried or chopped fresh mint until combined. Fold in drained cucumber. If desired, garnish with fresh mint leaves. If desired, serve with pitta bread or fresh vegetables. Cover and chill any remaining sauce for up to 24 hours.

Nutrition Facts per 115 g/4 oz: 49 cal., 2 g total fat (0 g sat. fat), 1 mg chol., 157 mg sodium, 5 g carbo., 0 g fibre, 3 g pro.

*Note: Be sure to use yogurt that contains no gums, gelatine, or fillers. These ingredients may prevent the curd and whey from separating to make the yogurt cheese.

**Note: If you are serving this as a dip, chop the cucumber slices after draining them on paper towels.

HARISSA
(TUNISIAN HOT CHILLI PASTE)

PREP: 25 MINUTES **STAND:** 1 HOUR **MAKES:** ABOUT 115 g/4 oz

4 dried guajillo chillies, stems and seeds removed*
5 dried ancho chillies, stems and seeds removed*
2 tablespoons extra-virgin olive oil
2 tablespoons water
2 cloves garlic, halved
2 teaspoons caraway seeds, toasted and ground, or 2 teaspoons caraway seeds, finely crushed**
1 teaspoon coriander seeds, toasted and ground, or ½ teaspoon ground coriander**
¼ teaspoon sea salt
⅛ teaspoon freshly ground black pepper

1. Heat a very large frying-pan over medium heat. Add dried chillies; toast for 2 minutes, turning occasionally. Place chillies in a very large bowl. Add enough boiling water to cover. Cover bowl and let stand for 1 hour. Drain well. Place chillies in a food processor; add oil, the 2 tablespoons water, the garlic, caraway seeds, coriander seeds, sea salt, and black pepper. Cover and process to a nearly smooth paste. Press mixture through a coarse-mesh strainer to remove chilli skins.

2. Transfer paste to a small bowl and use in recipes as directed. Use immediately or cover and chill for up to 2 weeks before using.

Nutrition Facts per tablespoon: 73 cal., 5 g total fat (0 g sat. fat), 0 mg chol., 71 mg sodium, 7 g carbo., 3 g fibre, 2 g pro.

*Note: Because chillies contain oils that can burn your skin and eyes, wear rubber or plastic gloves when working with them. If your bare hands do touch the chillies, wash your hands well with soap and water.

**Note: To toast seeds, heat a small frying-pan over medium heat. Add seeds. Cook about 2 minutes or until toasted and aromatic, shaking pan frequently. Place toasted seeds in a spice grinder and process until finely ground.

Harissa Sauce

START TO FINISH: 15 MINUTES **MAKES:** 170 g/6 oz

50 g/2 oz Harissa (Tunisian Hot Chilli Paste) (see recipe, page 141) or purchased
harissa
50 ml/2 fl oz water
 2 tablespoons extra-virgin olive oil
 2 tablespoons lemon juice
 1 teaspoon caraway seeds, toasted and ground,* or 1 teaspoon caraway seeds,
 finely crushed
 ½ teaspoon coriander seeds, toasted and ground,* or ¼ teaspoon ground
 coriander
 ¼ teaspoon sea salt
 ⅛ teaspoon freshly ground black pepper

1. In a small bowl whisk together Harissa, the water, oil, lemon juice, caraway seeds, coriander seeds, sea salt, and black pepper until combined. Serve with meat or fish, use as dip for whole wheat pitta bread, or add to Tunisian couscous.

Nutrition Facts per tablespoon: 46 cal., 4 g total fat (0 g sat. fat), 0 mg chol., 64 mg sodium, 3 g carbo., 1 g fibre, 1 g pro.

*Note: To toast seeds, heat a small frying-pan over medium heat. Add seeds. Cook about 2 minutes or until toasted and aromatic, shaking pan frequently. Place toasted seeds in a spice grinder and process until finely ground.

Cajun Beer Sauce

START TO FINISH: 15 MINUTES **MAKES:** 300 ml/½ pint

 40 g/1½ oz chopped onion
 50 g/2 oz chopped green or red pepper
 1 tablespoon extra-virgin olive oil
115 ml/4 fl oz beer
115 ml/4 fl oz water
 1 tablespoon cornflour
 1 tablespoon Cajun seasoning

1. In a small saucepan cook onion and pepper in hot oil until tender. In a small bowl stir together beer, the water, cornflour, and Cajun seasoning. Add to saucepan. Cook and stir over medium heat until thickened and bubbly. Cook and stir for 2 minutes more. Serve with grilled beef or lamb.

Nutrition Facts per tablespoon: 12 cal., 1 g total fat (0 g sat. fat), 0 mg chol., 28 mg sodium, 1 g carbo., 0 g fibre, 0 g pro.

TOMATO-WINE SAUCE

START TO FINISH: 15 MINUTES **MAKES:** 450 ml/³/₄ pint

70 g/2½ oz chopped onion
2 cloves garlic, minced
1 tablespoon extra-virgin olive oil
1 400 g/14 oz can chopped tomatoes, undrained
3 tablespoons dry white wine
1 tablespoon chopped fresh oregano or 1 teaspoon dried oregano, crushed
1 tablespoon capers, drained (optional)
⅛ teaspoon freshly ground black pepper

1. In a medium saucepan cook onion and garlic in hot oil until tender. Stir in undrained tomatoes, wine, oregano, capers (if desired), and black pepper. Bring to boiling; reduce heat. Simmer, uncovered, about 15 minutes or until desired consistency. Serve with grilled beef, pork, lamb, chicken, turkey, or fish.

Nutrition Facts per tablespoon: 9 cal., 0 g total fat (0 g sat. fat), 0 mg chol., 21 mg sodium, 1 g carbo., 0 g fibre, 0 g pro.

ONION SAUCE

START TO FINISH: 15 MINUTES **MAKES:** 300 ml/½ pint

225 g/8 oz chopped onions
1 clove garlic, minced
1 tablespoon extra-virgin olive oil
115 ml/4 fl oz dark beer or dark or amber non-alcoholic beer
115 ml/4 fl oz beef stock
1 tablespoon cornflour
1 tablespoon Worcestershire sauce

1. In a small saucepan cook onion and garlic in hot oil over medium heat about 4 minutes or until onions are tender. In a small bowl stir together beer, beef stock, cornflour, and Worcestershire sauce. Add to saucepan. Cook and stir over medium heat until thickened and bubbly. Cook and stir for 2 minutes more. Remove from heat. Serve with grilled beef, pork, or lamb.

Nutrition Facts per tablespoon: 14 cal., 1 g total fat (0 g sat. fat), 0 mg chol., 31 mg sodium, 2 g carbo., 0 g fibre, 0 g pro.

BASIL PESTO

START TO FINISH: 20 MINUTES **MAKES:** 115 g/4 oz

50 g/2 oz fresh basil leaves
25 g/1 oz pine nuts or almonds, toasted
3 tablespoons extra-virgin olive oil
2 cloves garlic, sliced
¼ teaspoon sea salt
⅛ teaspoon freshly ground black pepper
2 tablespoons finely shredded Parmesan cheese
1 to 2 tablespoons water (optional)

1. In a food processor combine basil, nuts, oil, garlic, sea salt, and black pepper. Cover and process until nearly smooth.

2. Transfer to a small bowl. Stir in cheese. If necessary, stir in enough of the water to make desired consistency. Serve immediately or cover the surface of the pesto with clingfilm to prevent browning and chill for up to 24 hours before serving.

Nutrition Facts per tablespoon: 79 cal., 8 g total fat (1 g sat. fat), 1 mg chol., 82 mg sodium, 1 g carbo., 0 g fibre, 2 g pro.

SPINACH PESTO WITH BALSAMIC VINEGAR

START TO FINISH: 20 MINUTES **MAKES:** 400 g/14 oz

50 ml/2 fl oz extra-virgin olive oil
4 cloves garlic, sliced
Dash sea salt
250 g/9 oz fresh spinach leaves
2 tablespoons balsamic vinegar
50 g/2 oz pine nuts or almonds, toasted
50 g/2 oz finely grated Parmesan cheese

1. In a medium frying-pan heat oil over medium-high heat just until hot. Stir in garlic and sea salt; remove from heat and set aside. In a large food processor combine spinach, vinegar, and nuts. Add oil mixture. Cover and process until nearly smooth. Stir in cheese. Use immediately or place in an airtight container and chill for up to 1 week or freeze in 1 tablespoon portions for up to 3 months before using. If frozen, thaw and stir before using.

Nutrition Facts per tablespoon: 42 cal., 4 g total fat (1 g sat. fat), 1 mg chol., 40 mg sodium, 1 g carbo., 0 g fibre, 2 g pro.

CRANBERRY-APPLE RELISH

PREP: 25 MINUTES **CHILL:** 24 HOURS TO 1 WEEK **MAKES:** 450 g/1 lb

2 apples, peeled, cored, and coarsely chopped
170 g/6 oz fresh cranberries
1 medium orange, peeled and sectioned
Dash ground cinnamon
Dash freshly ground black pepper
2 tablespoons honey
25 g/1 oz chopped walnuts, toasted

1. In a food processor combine apples, cranberries, orange sections, cinnamon, and black pepper. Cover and process until finely chopped.

2. Transfer the mixture to a medium saucepan. Stir in honey. Bring to boiling over medium-high heat; reduce heat. Simmer, uncovered, for 5 minutes, stirring frequently. Transfer to a medium bowl. Cover and chill for 24 hours to 1 week.

3. To serve, stir in walnuts. Serve on turkey, chicken, or ham sandwiches.

Nutrition Facts per 2 tablespoons: 37 cal., 1 g total fat (0 g sat. fat), 0 mg chol., 0 mg sodium, 7 g carbo., 1 g fibre, 0 g pro.

Spicy Fruit Salsa

PREP: 30 MINUTES **CHILL:** 15 MINUTES TO 24 HOURS
MAKES: 6 SERVINGS

50 g/2 oz chopped seeded, peeled fresh mango
50 g/2 oz chopped seeded, peeled fresh papaya
50 g/2 oz chopped cored, peeled fresh pineapple
40 g/1½ oz chopped red pepper
40 g/1½ oz chopped seeded fresh poblano chilli*
40 g/1½ oz chopped red onion
2 tablespoons chopped fresh coriander
1 tablespoon lime juice
2 teaspoons extra-virgin olive oil
1 teaspoon rice vinegar
½ of a medium fresh jalapeño chilli, seeded and finely chopped*
⅛ teaspoon sea salt

1. In a medium bowl combine mango, papaya, pineapple, pepper, poblano chilli, red onion, coriander, lime juice, oil, vinegar, jalapeño chilli, and sea salt. Stir gently to combine. Cover and chill for 15 minutes to 24 hours before serving. Serve with fish, pork, beef, chicken, or turkey.

Nutrition Facts per serving: 39 cal., 2 g total fat (0 g sat. fat), 0 mg chol., 42 mg sodium, 7 g carbo., 1 g fibre, 0 g pro.

*Note: Because chillies peppers contain oils that can burn your skin and eyes, wear rubber or plastic gloves when working with them. If your bare hands do touch the chillies, wash your hands well with soap and water.

BLUEBERRY SALSA

START TO FINISH: 20 MINUTES **MAKES:** 225 g/8 oz

170 g/6 oz fresh blueberries
2 oranges
40 g/1½ oz finely chopped red onion
2 tablespoons balsamic vinegar
1 tablespoon chopped fresh mint
¼ teaspoon sea salt

1. Coarsely chop 50 g/2 oz of the blueberries; add all of the blueberries to a medium bowl. Peel and section the oranges. Coarsely chop orange sections. Add chopped orange and any juice to the berries. Add red onion. Stir in balsamic vinegar, mint, and sea salt. Serve with grilled fish or chicken, or toss with mixed baby greens for a salad.

Nutrition Facts per 40 g/1½ oz: 46 cal., 0 g total fat (0 g sat. fat), 0 mg chol., 81 mg sodium, 11 g carbo., 2 g fibre, 1 g pro.

HUMMUS

START TO FINISH: 15 MINUTES **MAKES:** 400 g/14 oz

1 400 g/14 oz can chickpeas, rinsed and drained
50 g/2 oz tahini (sesame seed paste)
3 tablespoons water
2 tablespoons lemon juice
1 tablespoon extra-virgin olive oil
1 clove garlic, halved
½ teaspoon sea salt
½ teaspoon cumin seeds, toasted and ground,*
   or ½ teaspoon ground cumin
¼ teaspoon cayenne pepper
1 tablespoon chopped fresh flat-loaf parsley
Lemon juice (optional)
Fresh flat-leaf parsley

1. In a food processor combine chickpeas, beans, tahini, the water, the 2 tablespoons lemon juice, the oil, garlic, sea salt, cumin, and cayenne pepper. Cover and process until smooth. Transfer to a medium bowl. Stir in the 1 tablespoon parsley. If desired, stir in additional lemon juice to taste.

2. Garnish with additional parsley. Serve with baked pitta bread or crudités, or use as a spread in a grilled vegetable sandwich.

Nutrition Facts per 2 tablespoons: 71 cal., 4 g total fat (0 g sat. fat), 0 mg chol., 162 mg sodium, 8 g carbo., 2 g fibre, 2 g pro.

*Note: To toast seeds, heat a small frying-pan over medium heat. Add seeds. Cook about 2 minutes or until toasted and aromatic, shaking pan frequently. Place toasted seeds in a spice grinder and process until finely ground.

ROASTED GARLIC SPREAD

PREP: 10 MINUTES **ROAST:** 30 MINUTES (GARLIC) **OVEN:** 200°C/
400°F/gas mark 6 **MAKES:** 115 g/4 oz

**115 g/4 oz light mayonnaise or salad dressing
12 to 13 cloves (1 bulb) roasted garlic,* mashed**

1. In a small bowl stir together mayonnaise and garlic. Use immediately or cover and chill for up to 1 week before using. Use as a spread for sandwiches or wraps.

Nutrition Facts per tablespoon: 57 cal., 5 g total fat (1 g sat. fat), 5 mg chol., 91 mg sodium, 3 g carbo., 0 g fibre, 0 g pro.

*Note: To roast garlic, rub most of the papery skin off a bulb of garlic. With a sharp knife, slice off the top third of the garlic bulb to expose the cloves. Put garlic in a small baking dish and drizzle with about 1 teaspoon extra-virgin olive oil. Cover with foil. Roast in a 200°C/400°F/gas mark 6 oven for 30 to 35 minutes or until garlic is very tender. Squeeze the roasted garlic cloves into a small bowl and mash with a fork.

BLACK BEAN-SMOKED CHILLI SPREAD

START TO FINISH: 25 MINUTES **MAKES:** ABOUT 400 g/14 oz

70 g/2½ oz finely chopped onion
40 g/1½ oz sliced green onions
1 teaspoon ground coriander
1 teaspoon ground cumin
1 tablespoon extra-virgin olive oil
3 tablespoons chopped fresh coriander
1 × 400 g/14 oz tin black beans, rinsed and drained
115 ml/4 fl oz water
1 tablespoon lime juice
1 teaspoon finely chopped canned chipotle chilli in adobo sauce*
¼ teaspoon sea salt

1. In a covered small saucepan cook onions, coriander, and cumin in hot oil about 10 minutes or until very tender, stirring occasionally. Remove from heat; stir in coriander.

2. Transfer onion mixture to a blender or food processor. Add black beans, the water, lime juice, chilli, and sea salt. Cover and blend or process until nearly smooth. Serve immediately or cover and chill for up to 3 days before serving.

Nutrition Facts per tablespoon: 18 cal., 1 g total fat (0 g sat. fat), 0 mg chol., 61 mg sodium, 3 g carbo., 1 g fibre, 1 g pro.

*Note: Because hot chillies contain oils that can burn your skin and eyes, wear rubber or plastic gloves when working with them. If your bare hands do touch the chillies, wash your hands well with soap and water.

STANDARD VINAIGRETTE

START TO FINISH: 15 MINUTES **MAKES:** ABOUT 170 ml/6 fl oz

    50 ml/2 fl oz balsamic vinegar
     2 tablespoons finely chopped shallots
     1 clove garlic, minced
     1 tablespoon Dijon-style mustard
    115 ml/4 fl oz extra-virgin olive oil
     1 tablespoon chopped fresh flat-leaf parsley
     1 teaspoon chopped fresh thyme or ¼ teaspoon dried thyme, crushed
    ¼ teaspoon sea salt
     Dash freshly ground black pepper

1. In a medium bowl combine vinegar, shallots, and garlic. Let stand for 5 minutes. Whisk in mustard. Add oil in a thin, steady stream, whisking constantly until combined. Stir in parsley, thyme, sea salt, and black pepper. Use immediately or cover and chill for up to 3 days before using. If chilled, let stand at room temperature about 30 minutes; whisk before using.

Nutrition Facts per tablespoon: 90 cal., 9 g total fat (1 g sat. fat), 0 mg chol., 72 mg sodium, 2 g carbo., 0 g fibre, 0 g pro.

RED WINE VINAIGRETTE

START TO FINISH: 10 MINUTES **MAKES:** 85 ml/3 fl oz

     2 tablespoons red wine vinegar
     1 tablespoon finely chopped shallot
    1½ teaspoons Dijon-style mustard
     2 tablespoons extra-virgin olive oil
    ⅛ teaspoon sea salt
    ⅛ teaspoon freshly ground black pepper

1. In a small bowl combine vinegar and shallot. Let stand for 5 minutes. Whisk in mustard. Add oil in a thin, steady stream, whisking constantly until combined. Stir in sea salt and black pepper. Use immediately or cover and chill for up to 3 days before using. If chilled, let stand at room temperature about 30 minutes; whisk before using.

Nutrition Facts per tablespoon: 51 cal., 5 g total fat (1 g sat. fat), 0 mg chol., 85 mg sodium, 1 g carbo., 0 g fibre, 0 g pro.

LEMONY VINAIGRETTE

START TO FINISH: 15 MINUTES **MAKES:** ABOUT 170 ml/6 fl oz

50 ml/2 fl oz lemon juice
2 tablespoons finely chopped shallots
1 tablespoon water
1 clove garlic, minced
3 tablespoons extra-virgin olive oil
2 tablespoons chopped fresh herbs (such as oregano, rosemary, flat-leaf
  parsley, and/or thyme)
¼ teaspoon sea salt
¼ teaspoon freshly ground black pepper

1. In a small bowl combine lemon juice, shallots, the water, and garlic. Let stand for 5 minutes. Add oil in a thin, steady stream, whisking constantly until combined. Stir in herbs, sea salt, and black pepper. Use immediately or cover and chill for up to 3 days before using. If chilled, let stand at room temperature for 30 minutes; whisk before using.

Nutrition Facts per tablespoon: 40 cal., 4 g total fat (1 g sat. fat), 0 mg chol., 49 mg sodium, 1 g carbo., 0 g fibre, 0 g pro.

PEPPERCORN-STRAWBERRY VINAIGRETTE

START TO FINISH: 15 MINUTES **MAKES:** 150 ml/5 fl oz

150 g/5 oz cut-up fresh or frozen unsweetened strawberries, thawed
2 tablespoons red wine vinegar
Sugar substitute to equal ½ teaspoon sugar
¼ to ½ teaspoon cracked black pepper

1. In a blender combine strawberries, vinegar, sugar substitute, and black pepper. Cover and blend until smooth. Serve immediately or transfer to a storage container and cover and chill for up to 1 week.

Nutrition Facts per 2 tablespoons: 8 cal., 0 g total fat (0 g sat. fat), 0 mg chol., 0 mg sodium, 2 g carbo., 1 g fibre, 0 g pro.

GREEK VINAIGRETTE

START TO FINISH: 15 MINUTES **MAKES:** ABOUT 85 ml/3 fl oz

1 tablespoon red wine vinegar
1 tablespoon lemon juice
1 tablespoon finely chopped red onion
3 tablespoons extra-virgin olive oil
1 tablespoon chopped fresh mint
1 tablespoon chopped fresh oregano
   Dash sea salt
   Dash freshly ground black pepper

1. In a small bowl combine vinegar, lemon juice, and red onion. Let stand for 5 minutes. Add oil in a thin, steady stream, whisking constantly until combined. Stir in mint, oregano, sea salt, and black pepper. Use immediately or cover and chill for up to 3 days before using. If chilled, let stand at room temperature for 30 minutes; whisk before using.

Nutrition Facts per tablespoon: 73 cal., 8 g total fat (1 g sat. fat), 0 mg chol., 24 mg sodium, 0 g carbo., 0 g fibre, 0 g pro.

BALSAMIC VINAIGRETTE

START TO FINISH: 10 MINUTES **MAKES:** 225 ml/8 fl oz

115 ml/4 fl oz chicken stock or broth
 50 ml/2 fl oz balsamic vinegar
   1 tablespoon chopped fresh basil or 1 teaspoon dried basil, crushed
      Dash sea salt
 50 ml/2 fl oz extra-virgin olive oil
      Sea salt (optional)

1. In a small bowl combine chicken stock, vinegar, basil, and the dash sea salt. Add oil in a thin, steady stream, whisking constantly until combined. If desired, season to taste with additional sea salt. Use immediately or cover and chill for up to 1 week before using. If chilled, let stand at room temperature for 30 minutes; whisk before serving.

Nutrition Facts per tablespoon: 33 cal., 3 g total fat (0 g sat. fat), 0 mg chol., 38 mg sodium, 1 g carbo., 0 g fibre, 0 g pro.

Tip: For easy storage, combine the vinaigrette ingredients in a screw-top jar. Shake well before serving.

ASIAN-STYLE VINAIGRETTE

START TO FINISH: 10 MINUTES **MAKES:** ABOUT 170 ml/6 fl oz

50 ml/2 fl oz soy sauce
50 ml/2 fl oz lemon juice
1 tablespoon chopped fresh coriander
2 teaspoons grated fresh ginger
1 teaspoon honey
2 cloves garlic, minced
1 teaspoon toasted sesame oil

1. In a small bowl whisk together soy sauce, lemon juice, coriander, ginger, honey, garlic, and sesame oil until combined.

Nutrition Facts per tablespoon: 12 cal., 0 g total fat (0 g sat. fat), 0 mg chol., 412 mg sodium, 2 g carbo., 0 g fibre, 0 g pro.

PESTO VINAIGRETTE

START TO FINISH: 10 MINUTES **MAKES:** 170 ml/6 fl oz

50 g/2 oz packed fresh basil leaves
115 ml/4 fl oz extra-virgin olive oil
2 tablespoons pine nuts or walnuts, toasted
2 cloves garlic, minced
50 ml/2 fl oz white wine vinegar
½ teaspoon sea salt
¼ teaspoon freshly ground black pepper

1. In a food processor combine basil leaves, half the oil, the nuts, and garlic. Cover and pulse to a coarse purée. Transfer mixture to a small bowl. Whisk in remaining oil, the vinegar, sea salt, and black pepper.

Nutrition Facts per tablespoon: 92 cal., 10 g total fat (1 g sat. fat), 0 mg chol., 81 mg sodium, 1 g carbo., 0 g fibre, 1 g pro.

CREAMY ITALIAN DRESSING

START TO FINISH: 15 MINUTES **MAKES:** ABOUT 300 ml/½ pint

170 ml/6 fl oz low-fat soured cream or one 170 g/6 oz carton plain low-fat yogurt
50 ml/2 fl oz mayonnaise
2 teaspoons white wine vinegar or white vinegar
¼ teaspoon dry mustard
¼ teaspoon dried basil, crushed
¼ teaspoon dried oregano, crushed
⅛ teaspoon sea salt
⅛ teaspoon garlic powder
⅛ teaspoon freshly ground black pepper
85 to 115 ml/3 to 4 fl oz fat-free milk
Sea salt (optional)

1. In a small bowl whisk together soured cream, mayonnaise, vinegar, mustard, basil, oregano, the ⅛ teaspoon sea salt, the garlic powder, and black pepper. Whisk in enough of the milk to make desired consistency. If desired, season with additional sea salt.

2. Serve immediately or cover and chill for up to 1 week. Stir before serving. If necessary, stir in additional milk to make dressing of desired consistency.

Nutrition Facts per 2 tablespoons: 26 cal., 0 g total fat (0 g sat. fat), 0 mg chol., 112 mg sodium, 4 g carbo., 0 g fibre, 2 g pro.

Creamy Garlic Dressing: Prepare as above, except omit oregano and garlic powder. Add 2 cloves garlic, minced.

Nutrition Facts per 2 tablespoons: 26 cal., 0 g total fat (0 g sat. fat), 0 mg chol., 112 mg sodium, 4 g carbo., 0 g fibre, 2 g pro.

Creamy Parmesan Dressing: Prepare as above, except omit the dry mustard, dried oregano, and sea salt. Stir in 3 tablespoons grated Parmesan cheese and, if desired, use ½ teaspoon cracked black pepper in place of the ⅛ teaspoon freshly ground black pepper.

Nutrition Facts per 2 tablespoons: 32 cal., 0 g total fat (0 g sat. fat), 1 mg chol., 87 mg sodium, 4 g carbo., 0 g fibre, 2 g pro.

OIL-FREE HERB DRESSING

PREP: 15 MINUTES **CHILL:** 30 MINUTES **MAKES:** 115 ml/4 fl oz

1 tablespoon powdered fruit pectin
¾ teaspoon chopped fresh oregano, basil, thyme, tarragon, savory, or dill,
   or ¼ teaspoon dried, crushed
½ teaspoon sugar substitute (Splenda®)
⅛ teaspoon dry mustard
⅛ teaspoon freshly ground black pepper
¼ cup water
1 tablespoon white wine vinegar
1 small clove garlic, minced

1. In a small bowl stir together pectin, desired herb, sugar substitute, dry mustard, and black pepper. Stir in the water, vinegar, and garlic. Cover and chill for 30 minutes before serving. If desired, cover and store in the refrigerator for up to 3 days.

Nutrition Facts per 2 tablespoons: 17 cal., 0 g total fat (0 g sat. fat), 0 mg chol., 1 mg sodium, 4 g carbo., 0 g fibre, 0 g pro.

Oil-Free Creamy Onion Dressing: Prepare as above, except increase the sugar substitute to 1 tablespoon. Stir in 40 g/1½ oz thinly sliced spring onions and 50 g/2 oz plain low-fat yogurt with the water, vinegar, and garlic.

Nutrition Facts per 2 tablespoons: 19 cal., 0 g total fat (0 g sat. fat), 1 mg chol., 8 mg sodium, 4 g carbo., 0 g fibre, 1 g pro.

OIL-FREE FRENCH DRESSING

PREP: 10 MINUTES **CHILL:** 30 MINUTES **MAKES:** 225 ml/8 fl oz

    1 225 g/8 oz can tomato pasta sauce
    40 g/1½ oz chopped onion
    2 tablespoons cider vinegar
    2 teaspoons paprika
      Sugar substitute (Splenda®) equal to 2 teaspoons sugar
    ½ teaspoon garlic powder
    ⅛ teaspoon cayenne pepper

1. In a blender combine tomato sauce, onion, vinegar, paprika, sugar substitute, garlic powder, and cayenne pepper. Cover and blend until smooth. Transfer to a storage container; cover and chill for 30 minutes to blend flavours. Store any remaining dressing in the refrigerator for up to 2 days. If dressing is too thick, stir in enough water, 1 teaspoon at a time, to make desired consistency.

Nutrition Facts per per 2 tablespoons: 12 cal., 0 g total fat (0 g sat. fat), 0 mg chol., 131 mg sodium, 3 g carbo., 1 g fibre, 0 g pro.

SALSA DRESSING

START TO FINISH: 5 MINUTES **MAKES:** 170 ml/6 fl oz

50 g/2 oz plain fat-free yogurt
50 ml/2 fl oz low-fat soured cream
50 ml/2 fl oz bottled salsa
⅛ teaspoon sea salt
2 to 3 tablespoons fat-free milk

1. In a small bowl stir together yogurt, soured cream, salsa, and sea salt. Stir in enough of the milk to make desired consistency. Serve immediately or cover and chill up to 1 week.

Nutrition Facts per serving: 19 cal., 0 g total fat (0 g sat. fat), 0 mg chol.,
40 mg sodium, 3 g carbo., 0 g fibre, 1 g pro.

WAVE 1 MEAL PLANS

The meal plans that follow suggest exactly what to eat for breakfast, lunch, dinner, and snacks for each of the 10 days of Wave 1. As you use these menus, your meals will automatically conform to the Wave 1 guidelines. You'll also experience delicious new dishes that will actually increase your mealtime pleasure as you lose weight.

Instructions for preparing the main dishes for each meal are given in the Wave 1 recipe section. As with everything in the Sonoma Diet, the emphasis is on simplicity. All you have to do is fill the right-size plate with the Wave 1 proportions for each of the foods given. Then eat and enjoy.

Wave 1 is designed for fast initial weight loss as well as overcoming your sugar and refined grain cravings. These menus reflect the food choices that are part of Wave 1. For example, you'll find no fruits and only Tier 1 vegetables on any given day. The big plus of these menus is that they offer you tasty, satisfying meals .

But remember that these meal plans are optional. You can use them on all 10 days of Wave 1, on some of the days, or on none. You might find it convenient, for example, to follow the Wave 1 menus for most meals, but substitute a Sonoma Express recipe (see pages 127 and 128) when you're pressed for time. As long as your choices comform to the plate sizes and the Wave 1 proportions, you're home free. And throughout the day, don't forget to drink lots of water. It's especially important on this first part of the diet.

DAY ONE

Breakfast:	2 scrambled eggs with 1 slice whole grain toast
Lunch:	Greek Salad with Grilled Prawns (page 166) in ½ of a whole wheat pitta bread
Dinner:	Chicken en Papillote with Vegetables (page 167)
Snacks for Men:	33 almonds
Snacks for Women:	11 almonds

DAY TWO

Breakfast:	2 scrambled eggs with 1 slice whole grain toast
Lunch:	Chicken and Black Bean Wrap (page 168)
	Salad: 70 g / 2½ oz baby spinach, 1 tablespoon sliced almonds, Red Wine Vinaigrette (page 152)
Dinner:	Marinated Beef Steak (page 169)
	Sautéed Broccoli, Roasted Peppers, and Goat's Cheese (page 170)
Snacks for Men:	2 mozzarella string cheese sticks
	28 peanuts
Snacks for Women:	70 g / 2½ oz cherry tomatoes
	14 peanuts

DAY THREE

Breakfast: Mushroom Omelette (page 171)

Lunch: Steak and Blue Cheese Wrap (page 172)

Dinner: Mediterranean Pork Chops (page 173)

Broccoli with Almonds and Hot Pepper (page 174)

Toasted Quinoa Pilaf (page 175)

Snacks for Men: 22 almonds

Snacks for Women: 1 cucumber, sliced

70 g / 2½ oz raw pepper strips

DAY FOUR

Breakfast: 2 scrambled eggs with 1 slice whole grain toast

Lunch: Salad Niçoise with Tuna (page 176)

and ½ of a whole wheat wrap or pitta bread

Dinner: Tandoori Chicken (page 177)

Roasted Aubergine Salad (page 178)

Snacks for Men: 28 peanuts

cucumber or raw courgette slices topped with
3 Laughing Cow Light cheese spread triangles

Snacks for Women: 14 peanuts

cucumber or raw courgette slices topped with
1 Laughing Cow Light cheese spread triangle

DAY FIVE

Breakfast: Whole grain cereal with fat-free milk

Lunch: Grilled Asparagus Salad (page 179)

7 multigrain crackers or ½ of a whole wheat pitta bread

Dinner: Beef and Mushroom Kebabs (page 180)

Spinach salad with choice of vinaigrette

Snacks for Men: 1 Laughing Cow Mini Babybel cheese

150 g / 5 oz raw pepper strips

Snacks for Women: 1 Laughing Cow Mini Babybel cheese

150 g / 5 oz raw pepper strips

DAY SIX

Breakfast: Spanish Eggs (page 181)

Lunch: Mediterranean Tabbouleh Salad with Chicken (page 182)

Dinner: Easy Balsamic Chicken (page 183)

Roasted Vegetable Medley (page 184)

Snacks for Men: 22 almonds

2 tablespoons peanut butter on raw celery sticks

Snacks for Women: 11 almonds

1 tablespoon peanut butter on raw celery sticks

DAY SEVEN

Breakfast:	2 scrambled eggs with 1 slice whole grain toast
Lunch:	Chicken-Veggie Pitta Sandwich (page 185)
	150 g / 5 oz raw cauliflower, broccoli, and / or pepper strips
Dinner:	Sicilian Tuna Steak (page 186)
	Spinach salad with choice of vinaigrette
Snacks for Men:	22 almonds
	1 cucumber, cut into sticks
Snacks for Women:	70 g / 2½ oz cherry tomatoes
	1 cucumber, cut into sticks

DAY EIGHT

Breakfast:	Florentine Omelette (page 171)
Lunch:	Mediterranean Tuna and Caper Salad (page 187)
Dinner:	Roast Pork Loin with Vegetable Ratatouille (page 188) served over 50 g / 2 oz whole grain pasta
Snacks for Men:	2 mozzarella string cheese sticks
	28 peanuts
Snacks for Women:	50 g / 2 oz raw courgette sticks
	70 g / 2½ oz cherry tomatoes
	14 peanuts

DAY NINE

Breakfast:	Whole grain cereal with skimmed milk
Lunch:	Spinach and Lentil Salad with Toasted Walnuts (page 189)
Dinner:	Szechuan Prawns (page 190)
Snacks for Men:	22 almonds
	2 tablespoons peanut butter on raw celery sticks
Snacks for Women:	1 Laughing Cow Mini Babybel cheese
	1 tablespoon peanut butter on raw celery sticks

DAY TEN

Breakfast:	Baked Eggs (page 191)
Lunch:	Greek Chicken Salad with White Beans (page 192)
Dinner:	Halibut and Summer Vegetables en Papillote (page 193)
	70 g/2½ oz cooked brown rice
Snacks for Men:	3 Laughing Cow Mini Babybel cheeses
	22 almonds
	170 g/5 oz raw pepper strips
Snacks for Women:	1 Laughing Cow Mini Babybel cheese
	150 g/5 oz raw pepper strips

GREEK SALAD WITH GRILLED PRAWNS

PREP: 45 MINUTES **GRILL:** 6 MINUTES **MAKES:** 4 SERVINGS

450 g/1 lb fresh or frozen large prawns in shells
  2 cloves garlic, minced
  ½ teaspoon finely grated lemon peel
115 g/4 oz whole fresh baby spinach leaves
115 g/4 oz torn cos lettuce
  2 medium tomatoes, cut into thin wedges
  1 medium cucumber, quartered lengthwise and sliced 0.25 cm/¼ inch thick
40 g/1½ oz pitted kalamata olives
40 g/1½ oz chopped red onion
40 g/1½ oz thinly sliced radishes
25 g/1 oz crumbled feta cheese
  1 recipe Greek Vinaigrette
  2 large whole wheat pitta breads, halved crosswise

1. Thaw prawns, if frozen. Peel and devein prawns, leaving tails intact if desired. Rinse prawns; pat dry with paper towels. In a small bowl toss prawns with garlic and lemon peel. Cover and chill for 30 minutes.

2. Meanwhile, in a large bowl combine spinach, lettuce, tomatoes, cucumber, olives, red onion, and radishes; toss to combine. Set aside.

3. Thread prawns onto four 20-cm/8-inch skewers,* leaving a 0.5-cm/¼-inch space between pieces.

4. Place skewers on the greased rack of a grill or barbecue and grill for 6 to 8 minutes or until prawns are opaque, turning once halfway through grilling.

5. To serve, divide greens mixture among 4 dinner plates. Sprinkle with feta cheese. Top with grilled prawns. Drizzle with Greek Vinaigrette. Serve with pitta bread.

Greek Vinaigrette: In a screw-top jar combine 3 tablespoons extra-virgin olive oil, 1 tablespoon red wine vinegar, 1 tablespoon lemon juice, 1 tablespoon chopped fresh mint, 1 tablespoon chopped fresh oregano, dash sea salt, and dash freshly ground black pepper. Cover and shake well.

Nutrition Facts per serving: 369 cal., 16 g total fat (3 g sat. fat), 179 mg chol., 571 mg sodium, 29 g carbo., 6 g fibre, 30 g pro.

*Note: If using wooden skewers, soak in enough water to cover for at least 1 hour before grilling.

Chicken en Papillote with Vegetables

PREP: 35 MINUTES **BAKE:** 20 MINUTES **OVEN:** 200°C/400°F/GAS MARK 6 **MAKES:** 4 SERVINGS

450 g/1 lb skinless, boneless chicken breast halves
2 tablespoons extra-virgin olive oil
1 tablespoon chopped fresh oregano or 1 teaspoon dried oregano, crushed
1 tablespoon chopped fresh thyme or ½ teaspoon dried thyme, crushed
1 teaspoon finely shredded lemon peel
2 tablespoons lemon juice
½ teaspoon sea salt
¼ teaspoon freshly ground black pepper
275 g/10 oz fresh asparagus, trimmed and cut into 5-cm/2-inch pieces
170 g/6 oz mangetout peas, trimmed
4 canned artichoke hearts, drained and quartered, or 4 frozen artichoke hearts, thawed and quartered
150 g/5 oz cherry tomatoes, halved
2 tablespoons chopped fresh flat-leaf parsley
Parchment paper
70 g/2½ oz sliced spring onions

1. Cut chicken breasts crosswise into 1-cm/½-inch slices. In a medium bowl combine oil, oregano, thyme, lemon peel, lemon juice, sea salt, and black pepper. Add chicken to bowl and toss to coat. Let stand while preparing vegetables.

2. In a large bowl combine asparagus, mangetout, artichoke hearts, cherry tomatoes, and parsley. Tear four 20×5-cm/2-inch pieces of parchment paper; fold each in half crosswise and crease. Open up again. On half of one parchment sheet, arrange one quarter of the vegetable mixture. Top with one quarter of the chicken pieces. Top with quarter of the spring onions. To make packet, fold parchment paper over chicken and vegetables. Crimp and fold edges to seal; twist corners. Repeat to make 4 packets.

3. Place 2 packets on each of 2 baking sheets. Bake on separate racks in a 200°C/400°F/gas mark 6 oven about 20 minutes or until chicken is no longer pink. (To test, carefully open the packets and peek.) Serve immediately.

Nutrition Facts per serving: 249 cal., 8 g total fat (1 g sat. fat), 66 mg chol., 498 mg sodium, 13 g carbo., 6 g fibre, 31 g pro.

CHICKEN AND BLACK BEAN WRAP

START TO FINISH: 10 MINUTES **MAKES:** 1 SERVING

- 2 tablespoons Black Bean-Smoked Chilli Spread (see recipe, page 151)
- 1 20-cm/8-inch whole wheat flour tortilla
- 85 g/3 oz chopped cooked skinless chicken or turkey breast
- 40 g/1½ oz shredded or torn cos lettuce or whole fresh baby spinach leaves
- 3 tablespoons chopped fresh coriander
- 1 tablespoon bottled salsa

1. Place spread on one side of the tortilla. Top with chicken, lettuce, coriander, and salsa. Roll up.

Nutrition Facts per serving: 322 cal., 8 g total fat (2 g sat. fat), 72 mg chol., 554 mg sodium, 24 g carbo., 14 g fibre, 38 g pro.

MARINATED BEEF STEAK

PREP: 20 MINUTES **MARINATE:** 1 TO 24 HOURS **GRILL:** 17 MINUTES
STAND: 10 MINUTES **MAKES:** 8 SERVINGS

1 675 to 900 g/1½ to 2 lb beef steak
3 tablespoons chopped fresh rosemary or 1 tablespoon dried rosemary,
   crushed
1 tablespoon chopped fresh marjoram or 1 teaspoon dried marjoram, crushed
1 tablespoon chopped fresh oregano or 1 teaspoon dried oregano, crushed
3 cloves garlic, minced
1½ teaspoons paprika
1 teaspoon sea salt
1 teaspoon crushed red pepper
1 teaspoon freshly ground black pepper
3 tablespoons extra-virgin olive oil

1. Trim fat from meat. Score both sides of steak in a diamond pattern by making shallow cuts at 2.5-cm/1-inch intervals; set aside. In a small bowl stir together rosemary, marjoram, oregano, garlic, paprika, sea salt, crushed red pepper, and black pepper. Stir in the oil until combined.

2. Spoon herb mixture evenly over both sides of steak; rub in with your fingers. Place steak in a shallow dish. Cover and marinate in the refrigerator for 1 to 24 hours.

3. Place meat on the rack of a grill or barbecue and grill for 17 to 21 minutes or until medium doneness, turning once halfway through grilling.

4. Transfer meat to a cutting board. Cover and let stand for 10 minutes. To serve, slice very thinly across the grain.

Nutrition Facts per serving: 183 cal., 11 g total fat (3 g sat. fat), 34 mg chol., 287 mg sodium, 1 g carbo., 0 g fibre, 19 g pro.

Sautéed Broccoli, Roasted Peppers, and Goat's Cheese

START TO FINISH: 30 MINUTES **MAKES:** 4 SERVINGS

2 tablespoons extra-virgin olive oil
450 g/1 lb broccoli florets
2 cloves garlic, thinly sliced
115 g/4 oz bottled roasted red peppers, drained and chopped
40 g/1½ oz chopped, pitted kalamata olives
2 tablespoons chopped fresh flat-leaf parsley
1 spring onion, thinly sliced
1 tablespoon chopped fresh marjoram or 1 teaspoon dried marjoram, crushed
1 tablespoon lemon juice
¼ teaspoon sea salt
⅛ teaspoon freshly ground black pepper
50 g/2 oz goat's cheese, crumbled

1. In a large frying-pan heat oil over medium heat. Add broccoli and garlic; cook for 5 to 8 minutes or until broccoli is crisp-tender. Stir in roasted peppers, olives, parsley, spring onion, marjoram, lemon juice, sea salt, and black pepper. Heat through. Transfer mixture to 4 serving plates or a platter; sprinkle with goat's cheese.

Nutrition Facts per serving: 167 cal., 12 g total fat (4 g sat. fat), 11 mg chol., 299 mg sodium, 11 g carbo., 4 g fibre, 6 g pro.

MUSHROOM OMELETTE

START TO FINISH: 20 MINUTES **MAKES:** 1 SERVING

2 eggs
⅛ teaspoon sea salt
⅛ teaspoon freshly ground black pepper
2 teaspoons olive oil
50 g/2 oz sliced fresh mushrooms

1. In a small bowl beat eggs, sea salt, and black pepper with a whisk until combined; set aside. In a medium non-stick frying-pan with flared sides heat 1 teaspoon of the oil over medium heat. Add mushrooms; cook until tender, stirring occasionally. Remove mushrooms from pan; set aside.

2. Add remaining 1 teaspoon oil to same pan. Heat over medium heat. Add egg mixture to pan. Immediately begin stirring egg mixture gently but continuously with a wooden or plastic spatula until mixture resembles small pieces of cooked egg surrounded by liquid egg. Stop stirring. Cook for 30 to 60 seconds more or until egg mixture is set but shiny.

3. Sprinkle mushrooms across centre of the egg mixture. With a spatula, lift and fold an edge of the omelette about a third of the way towards the centre. Remove from heat. Fold the opposite edge toward the centre; transfer to a warm plate, seam side down.

Nutrition Facts per serving: 236 cal., 19 g total fat (4 g sat. fat), 423 mg chol., 383 mg sodium, 2 g carbo., 0 g fibre, 14 g pro.

Ranchero Omelette: Prepare as above, except omit mushrooms and 1 teaspoon of the oil. Top cooked egg mixture with 1 tablespoon chopped red, green, or yellow pepper; 1 tablespoon chopped tomato; 1 tablespoon grated Monterey Jack or Cheddar cheese; ½ teaspoon chopped fresh coriander; and ¼ teaspoon finely chopped, seeded fresh jalapeño or serrano chilli* before folding.

Nutrition Facts per serving: 219 cal., 17 g total fat (5 g sat. fat), 429 mg chol., 420 mg sodium, 2 g carbo., 0 g fibre, 15 g pro.

Florentine Omelette: Prepare as above, except omit mushrooms and 1 teaspoon of the oil. Sprinkle cooked egg mixture with 1 teaspoon chopped fresh dill or ¼ teaspoon dried dill; top with 50 g/2 oz frozen chopped spinach, thawed and well drained, and 1 tablespoon shredded Swiss cheese before folding.

Nutrition Facts per serving: 231 cal., 17 g total fat (5 g sat. fat), 430 mg chol., 426 mg sodium, 3 g carbo., 1 g fibre, 16 g pro.

*Note: Because chillies contain oils that can burn your skin and eyes, wear rubber or plastic gloves when working with them. If your bare hands do touch the chillies, wash your hands well with soap and water.

STEAK AND BLUE CHEESE WRAP

START TO FINISH: 10 MINUTES **MAKES:** 1 SERVING

85 g/3 oz leftover grilled Marinated Beef Steak (see recipe, page 169), thinly sliced
40 g/1½ oz shredded cos lettuce or whole fresh baby spinach leaves
25 g/1 oz bottled roasted red peppers, drained and cut into thin strips
 1 tablespoon crumbled blue cheese
 1 20-cm/8-inch whole wheat flour tortilla

1. Arrange sliced beef, lettuce, roasted pepper strips, and blue cheese on top of the tortilla. Roll up (tortilla will be very full).

Nutrition Facts per serving: 390 cal., 19 g total fat (6 g sat. fat), 46 mg chol., 775 mg sodium, 21 g carbo., 13 g fibre, 33 g pro.

MEDITERRANEAN PORK CHOPS

PREP: 10 MINUTES **ROAST:** 35 MINUTES **OVEN:** 220°C/425°F/
GAS MARK 7, REDUCING TO 180°C/350°F/GAS MARK 4
MAKES: 4 SERVINGS

- 4 boneless or bone-in pork loin chops, cut 1 cm/½ inch thick (450 to 675 g/
  1 to 1½ lb)
- ½ teaspoon sea salt
- ¼ teaspoon freshly ground black pepper
- 1 tablespoon finely chopped fresh rosemary or 1 teaspoon dried rosemary,
  crushed
- 3 cloves garlic, minced

1. Sprinkle chops with sea salt and black pepper; set aside. In a small bowl combine rosemary and garlic. Sprinkle rosemary mixture evenly over both sides of each chop; rub in with your fingers.

2. Place chops on a rack in a shallow roasting pan. Roast chops in a 220°C/425°F/gas mark 7 oven for 10 minutes. Reduce oven temperature to 180°C/350°F/gas mark 4 and continue roasting about 25 minutes.

Nutrition Facts per serving: 147 cal., 4 g total fat (2 g sat. fat), 71 mg chol., 288 mg sodium, 1 g carbo., 0 g fibre, 24 g.

BROCCOLI WITH ALMONDS AND HOT PEPPER

START TO FINISH: 15 MINUTES **MAKES:** 4 SERVINGS

- 450 g/1 lb broccoli florets
- 4 cloves garlic, minced
- 2 tablespoons extra-virgin olive oil
- 1 tablespoon lemon juice
- 25 g/1 oz sliced almonds, toasted
- ¼ to ½ teaspoon crushed red pepper
- ¼ teaspoon sea salt

1. In a large frying-pan cook broccoli and garlic in hot oil over medium heat for 5 to 8 minutes or until broccoli is crisp-tender. Stir in lemon juice. Sprinkle with almonds, crushed red pepper, and sea salt; toss to combine.

Nutrition Facts per serving: 142 cal., 11 g total fat (1 g sat. fat), 0 mg chol., 150 mg sodium, 9 g carbo., 3 g fibre, 4 g pro.

TOASTED QUINOA PILAF

PREP: 20 MINUTES **COOK:** 20 MINUTES **MAKES:** 12 SERVINGS

2 tablespoons finely chopped shallots or onion
6 cloves garlic, minced
1 tablespoon extra-virgin olive oil
400 g/14 oz quinoa,* or barley, rinsed and well drained
700 ml/1¼ pints chicken stock
1½ teaspoons chopped fresh thyme or ½ teaspoon dried thyme, crushed
1 bay leaf
115 g/4 oz bottled roasted red peppers, diced
Sea salt
Freshly ground black pepper

1. In a large saucepan cook shallots and garlic in hot oil over medium heat until tender. Carefully stir in quinoa or barley. Cook and stir about 5 minutes or until quinoa or barley is golden brown. Carefully stir in stock, thyme, and bay leaf. Bring to boiling; reduce heat. Cover and simmer about 20 minutes or until quinoa is tender and fluffy (cook barley about 10 minutes or until tender and liquid is absorbed).

2. Discard bay leaf. Gently stir in roasted peppers. Season to taste with sea salt and black pepper.

Nutrition Facts per serving: 125 cal., 3 g total fat (0 g sat. fat), 0 mg chol., 169 mg sodium, 21 g carbo., 2 g fibre, 4 g pro.

*Note: Look for quinoa at a health food shop or in the grains section of a large supermarket.

Salad Niçoise with Tuna

START TO FINISH: 35 MINUTES **MAKES:** 4 SERVINGS

115 g/4 oz green beans
170 g/6 oz torn mixed salad greens
    1 170 g/6 oz can tuna (water pack), drained and broken into chunks
    4 medium tomatoes, quartered
    2 hard-boiled eggs, peeled and quartered
    6 tablespoons chopped fresh flat-leaf parsley
    3 spring onions, cut into 0.25 cm/½-inch slices
    4 anchovy fillets, drained, rinsed, and patted dry (optional)
125 g/4½ oz pitted ripe olives
    1 recipe Niçoise Dressing

1. Wash green beans; remove ends and strings. Leave beans whole or snap in half. In a covered medium saucepan cook green beans in a small amount of boiling lightly salted water for 5 minutes or just until tender. Drain and place in ice water until chilled; drain well. If desired, cover and chill for 2 to 24 hours.

2. Line a large platter or 4 serving plates with salad greens. Arrange green beans, tuna, tomatoes, and eggs on the greens. Sprinkle with parsley and spring onions. If desired, top with anchovy fillets. Top with olives. Drizzle Niçoise Dressing over all.

Niçoise Dressing: In a small bowl combine 3 tablespoons extra-virgin olive oil, 1 tablespoon white wine vinegar, ½ teaspoon Dijon-style mustard, ¼ teaspoon sea salt, and ⅛ teaspoon freshly ground black pepper. Whisk together until combined.

Nutrition Facts per serving: 260 cal., 17 g total fat (3 g sat. fat), 124 mg chol., 570 mg sodium, 12 g carbo., 5 g fibre, 16 g pro.

TANDOORI CHICKEN

PREP: 20 MINUTES **CHILL:** 24 TO 48 HOURS
MARINATE: 1 TO 3 HOURS **GRILL:** 10 MINUTES **MAKES:** 4 SERVINGS

115 g/4 oz plain fat-free yogurt*
  4 skinless, boneless chicken breast halves (450 to 565 g/1 to 1¼ lb total)
⅛ teaspoon sea salt
⅛ teaspoon freshly ground black pepper
50 ml/2 fl oz lemon juice
  3 cloves garlic, minced
  2 teaspoons paprika
¼ teaspoon cayenne pepper
⅛ teaspoon ground cinnamon
⅛ teaspoon ground cumin

1. To make yogurt cheese, line a yogurt strainer, sieve, or small colander with three layers of 100% cotton cheesecloth or a clean paper coffee filter. Suspend lined strainer, sieve, or colander over a bowl. Spoon yogurt into lined strainer, sieve, or colander. Cover with plastic wrap. Refrigerate for 24 to 48 hours. Discard liquid.

2. Sprinkle chicken with sea salt and black pepper. Place chicken in a self-sealing plastic bag set in a shallow dish. In a small bowl combine the yogurt cheese, lemon juice, garlic, paprika, cayenne pepper, cinnamon, and cumin. Pour over chicken. Cover and marinate in the refrigerator for 1 to 3 hours.

3. Remove chicken from marinade and discard any remaining marinade. Place chicken on the rack of a grill or barbecue and grill for 10 to 12 minutes or until chicken is no longer pink, turning once halfway through grilling.

Nutrition Facts per serving: 152 cal., 2 g total fat (0 g sat. fat), 66 mg chol., 144 mg sodium, 5 g carbo., 1 g fibre, 28 g pro.

*Note: Be sure to use yogurt that contains no gums, gelatine, or fillers. These ingredients may prevent the curd and whey from separating to make the yogurt cheese.

Tip: If you want leftover chicken to use for another meal, double this recipe.

ROASTED AUBERGINE SALAD

PREP: 40 MINUTES **STAND:** 20 MINUTES **BAKE:** 20 MINUTES
OVEN: 200°C/400°F/GAS MARK 6 **MAKES:** 8 SERVINGS

Non-stick olive oil cooking spray
2 aubergines, peeled, if desired, and cut crosswise into 2.5-cm/1-inch slices
(about 1.1 kg/2½ lb)
1 teaspoon sea salt
2 cloves garlic, minced
1 tablespoon chopped fresh oregano or 1 teaspoon dried oregano, crushed
¼ teaspoon freshly ground black pepper
2 tablespoons extra-virgin olive oil
2 tablespoons red wine vinegar
1 tablespoon water
1½ teaspoons chopped fresh marjoram or ½ teaspoon dried marjoram, crushed
⅛ teaspoon freshly ground black pepper
1 red onion, sliced 1 cm/½ inch thick
115 g/4 oz bottled roasted red peppers, drained and chopped
6 tablespoons fresh flat-leaf parsley leaves
2 tablespoons capers, rinsed and drained
2 tablespoons chopped pitted kalamata olives
2 tablespoons lemon juice
225 g/8 oz whole fresh baby spinach leaves
25 g/1 oz crumbled feta cheese

1. Lightly coat a baking sheet with non-stick cooking spray. Arrange aubergine slices on baking sheet. Sprinkle with ½ teaspoon of the sea salt. Let stand for 20 minutes. Place aubergine slices in a colander; rinse with cold water and drain well. Pat dry with paper towels. Arrange on the same baking sheet. Sprinkle with garlic, oregano, ¼ teaspoon of the sea salt, and ¼ teaspoon black pepper. Drizzle with 1 tablespoon of the oil. Bake, uncovered, in a 200°C/400°F/gas mark 6 oven about 15 minutes or just until tender, turning once. Cool slightly and cut into 2.5-cm/1-inch cubes.

2. Meanwhile, in a 2.2-litre/4-pint square baking dish combine remaining 1 tablespoon oil, 1 tablespoon of the red wine vinegar, the water, marjoram, remaining ¼ teaspoon sea salt, and the ⅛ teaspoon black pepper. Add red onion slices; turn several times to coat. Bake, covered, in the 200°C/400°F/gas mark 6 oven about 20 minutes or until tender, turning onion slices once. Cool slightly in dish on wire rack. Chop the onion, reserving any liquid in the dish.

3. In a large bowl combine aubergine, onion, roasted peppers, parsley leaves, capers, olives, lemon juice, and remaining 1 tablespoon red wine vinegar.

4. Arrange spinach leaves on a large platter or on 8 serving plates. Top with aubergine mixture. Sprinkle with feta cheese and drizzle with reserved liquid from dish.

Nutrition Facts per serving: 97 cal., 5 g total fat (1 g sat. fat), 3 mg chol., 270 mg sodium, 13 g carbo., 7 g fibre, 3 g pro.

GRILLED ASPARAGUS SALAD

PREP: 15 MINUTES **GRILL:** 5 MINUTES **MAKES:** 2 SERVINGS

340 g/12 oz fresh asparagus (thick spears), trimmed
1 tablespoon extra-virgin olive oil
¼ teaspoon sea salt
⅛ teaspoon freshly ground black pepper
3 tablespoons lemon juice
1 tablespoon extra-virgin olive oil
2 hard-boiled eggs, peeled and chopped
1 tablespoon grated Parmesan cheese

1. In a large bowl toss asparagus spears with 1 tablespoon olive oil. Sprinkle with sea salt and black pepper.

2. Place asparagus spears crosswise on the rack of a grill or barbecue and grill for 5 to 7 minutes or until asparagus is crisp-tender and slightly charred all over, turning occasionally.

3. To serve, transfer grilled asparagus to serving platter. Drizzle with lemon juice and 1 tablespoon olive oil. Sprinkle with chopped eggs and Parmesan cheese. Serve immediately or cover and chill for up to 24 hours.

Nutrition Facts per serving: 247 cal., 20 g total fat (4 g sat. fat), 214 mg chol., 350 mg sodium, 9 g carbo., 4 g fibre, 11 g pro.

BEEF AND MUSHROOM KEBABS

PREP: 25 MINUTES **MARINATE:** 30 MINUTES TO 1 HOUR
GRILL: 8 MINUTES **MAKES:** 6 SERVINGS

85 ml/3 fl oz balsamic vinegar
2 tablespoons extra-virgin olive oil
2 tablespoons water
1 medium shallot, thinly sliced
2 tablespoons chopped fresh oregano or 2 teaspoons dried oregano, crushed
1½ teaspoons chopped fresh thyme or ½ teaspoon dried thyme, crushed
2 cloves garlic, minced
¾ teaspoon sea salt
½ teaspoon freshly ground black pepper
675 g/1½ lb beef steak or sirloin, cut into 2.5-cm/1-inch cubes
Sea salt
Freshly ground black pepper
225 g/8 oz fresh mushrooms
12 cherry tomatoes

1. For marinade, in a medium bowl combine vinegar, oil, the water, shallot, oregano, thyme, garlic, the ¾ teaspoon sea salt, and the ½ teaspoon black pepper.

2. Season meat with additional sea salt and black pepper. Place meat in a self-sealing plastic bag set in a shallow dish. Pour half of the marinade over meat. (Reserve remaining marinade for vegetables.) Seal bag; turn to coat meat. Marinate meat in refrigerator for 30 minutes to 1 hour, turning bag occasionally.

3. Place mushrooms and cherry tomatoes in another self-sealing plastic bag set in a shallow dish. Pour remaining marinade over vegetables. Seal bag; turn to coat vegetables. Marinate at room temperature for 20 minutes.

4. Drain meat and vegetables, discarding marinade. On twelve 25-cm/10-inch skewers,* alternately thread beef, mushrooms, and tomatoes, leaving a 0.5-cm/¼-inch space between pieces.

5. Place kebabs on the rack of a grill or barbecue and grill until desired doneness, turning kebabs once halfway through grilling. Allow 8 to 12 minutes for medium-rare doneness or 12 to 15 minutes for medium doneness.

Nutrition Facts per serving: 220 cal., 11 g total fat (4 g sat. fat), 70 mg chol., 177 mg sodium, 4 g carbo., 1 g fibre, 25 g pro.

*Note: If using wooden skewers, soak them in water at least 1 hour before using.

SPANISH EGGS

START TO FINISH: 30 MINUTES **MAKES:** 4 SERVINGS

    1 yellow pepper, cut into thin bite-size strips
    1 fresh jalapeño chilli, seeded and chopped*
    2 cloves garlic, minced
    1 tablespoon extra-virgin olive oil
600 g/1 lb 6 oz tomatoes, seeded and chopped
    1 to 1½ teaspoons chilli powder
    ½ teaspoon ground cumin
    ¼ teaspoon sea salt
    4 eggs
      Sea salt
      Freshly ground black pepper
    2 tablespoons sliced almonds, toasted

1. In a large frying-pan cook pepper, chilli, and garlic in hot oil about 2 minutes or until tender. Stir in tomatoes, chilli powder, cumin, and the ¼ teaspoon sea salt. Bring to boiling; reduce heat. Cover and simmer for 5 minutes.

2. Break one of the eggs into a cup. Carefully slide the egg into simmering tomato mixture. Repeat with remaining eggs. Sprinkle eggs lightly with additional sea salt and black pepper.

3. Cook, covered, over medium-low heat for 4 to 5 minutes or until whites are completely set and yolks begin to thicken but are not firm.

4. To serve, transfer eggs to serving plates with a slotted spoon. Stir tomato mixture; spoon around eggs on plates. Sprinkle with toasted almonds.

Nutrition Facts per serving: 173 cal., 11 g total fat (2 g sat. fat), 212 mg chol., 267 mg sodium, 11 g carbo., 3 g fibre, 9 g pro.

*Note: Because chillies contain oils that can burn your skin and eyes, wear rubber or plastic gloves when working with them. If your bare hands do touch the chillies, wash your hands well with soap and water.

Mediterranean Tabbouleh Salad with Chicken

PREP: 30 MINUTES **STAND:** 30 MINUTES **CHILL:** 4 TO 24 HOURS
MAKES: 6 SERVINGS

340 ml/12 fl oz water
90 g/3½ oz bulgur
2 medium tomatoes, chopped
1 cup finely chopped, seeded cucumber
50 g/2 oz finely chopped flat-leaf parsley
50 g/2 oz thinly sliced spring onions
3 tablespoons chopped fresh mint or 1 tablespoon dried mint, crushed
85 to 115 ml/3 to 4 fl oz lemon juice
50 ml/2 fl oz extra-virgin olive oil
¾ teaspoon sea salt
½ teaspoon freshly ground black pepper
12 large cos lettuce leaves
500 g/1 lb 2 oz grilled skinless, boneless chicken breast halves,* sliced

1. In a large bowl combine the water and bulgur. Let stand for 30 minutes. Drain bulgur through a fine sieve, using a large spoon to push out excess water. Return bulgur to bowl. Stir in tomatoes, cucumber, parsley, spring onions, and mint.

2. For dressing, in a screw-top jar combine lemon juice, oil, sea salt, and black pepper. Cover and shake well. Pour dressing over the bulgur mixture. Toss lightly to coat. Cover and chill for 4 to 24 hours, stirring occasionally. Bring to room temperature before serving.

3. For each serving, place 2 lettuce leaves on a serving plate. Top each with 115 g/4 oz of the bulgur mixture and 85 g/3 oz of the cooked chicken.

Nutrition Facts per serving: 298 cal., 13 g total fat (2 g sat. fat), 72 mg chol., 324 mg sodium, 17 g carbo., 5 g fibre, 30 g pro.

*Note: To grill chicken breast halves, lightly sprinkle chicken with sea salt and freshly ground black pepper. Place chicken on the rack of a grill or barbecue and grill for 10 to 12 minutes or until chicken is no longer pink, turning once halfway through grilling.

EASY BALSAMIC CHICKEN

PREP: 15 MINUTES **MARINATE:** 1 TO 4 HOURS **GRILL:** 10 MINUTES
MAKES: 4 SERVINGS

  4 skinless, boneless chicken breast halves (450 to 565 g/1 to 1¼ lb pounds
    total)
50 ml/2 fl oz balsamic vinegar
50 ml/2 fl oz olive oil
  3 cloves garlic, minced
¼ teaspoon sea salt
¼ teaspoon crushed red pepper

1. Place each chicken breast between 2 pieces of clingfilm. Using the flat side of a meat mallet, pound lightly to 1-cm/½ inch thickness. Remove clingfilm.

2. Place chicken in a self-sealing plastic bag. In a small bowl combine vinegar, oil, garlic, sea salt, and crushed red pepper. Pour over chicken. Seal bag; turn to coat chicken. Cover and marinate in the refrigerator for 1 to 4 hours, turning bag occasionally.

3. Drain, discarding marinade. Place chicken on the rack of a grill or barbecue and grill for 10 to 12 minutes or until chicken is no longer pink, turning once halfway through grilling.

Nutrition Facts per serving: 177 cal., 6 g total fat (2 g sat. fat), 66 mg chol., 125 mg sodium, 2 g carbo., 0 g fibre, 26 g pro.

Oven method: Place chicken on a rack in a shallow roasting pan. Roast chicken in a 200°C/400°F/gas mark 6 oven for about 15 minutes or until chicken is no longer pink.

ROASTED VEGETABLE MEDLEY

PREP: 25 MINUTES **BAKE:** 35 MINUTES **OVEN:** 200°C/400°F/
GAS MARK 6 **MAKES:** 4 SERVINGS

225 g/8 oz Brussels sprouts
225 g/8 oz green beans, cut into 5-cm/2-inch pieces
225 g/8 oz cauliflower florets
  2 tablespoons chopped fresh herbs or 2 teaspoons dried herbs, crushed (such as rosemary, basil, and oregano)
  ¼ teaspoon sea salt
  ⅛ teaspoon freshly ground black pepper
  2 tablespoons extra-virgin olive oil
  2 tablespoons water
  3 red, yellow, and/or green peppers, seeded and cut into strips

1. Halve any large Brussels sprouts. Place Brussels sprouts, green beans, and cauliflower in a shallow roasting pan. Sprinkle with desired herbs, sea salt, and black pepper. Drizzle with oil and the water.

2. Cover with foil. Bake in a 200°C/400°F/gas mark 6 oven for 20 minutes. Remove foil; stir in peppers. Bake, uncovered, about 15 minutes more or until vegetables are crisp-tender.

Nutrition Facts per serving: 129 cal., 7 g total fat (1 g sat. fat), 0 mg chol., 152 mg sodium, 15 g carbo., 7 g fibre, 5 g pro.

CHICKEN-VEGGIE PITTA SANDWICH

START TO FINISH: 20 MINUTES **MAKES:** 2 SERVINGS

1 large whole wheat pitta bread
115 g/4 oz assorted fresh vegetables (such as bite-size red or yellow pepper
   strips, coarsely chopped broccoli or cauliflower florets, chopped courgettes
   or yellow pattypan squash, and/or chopped, seeded cucumber)
50 g/2 oz Yogurt and Cucumber Sauce (see recipe, page 140)
115 g/4 oz cooked skinless chicken breast, sliced

1. Cut pitta bread in half crosswise. Carefully split each half open to form a pocket. In a small bowl toss vegetables and Yogurt and Cucumber Sauce together. Spoon into pitta halves. Add half of the chicken to each pitta pocket.

Nutrition Facts per serving: 220 cal., 4 g total fat (1 g sat. fat), 49 mg chol., 296 mg sodium, 23 g carbo., 3 g fibre, 23 g pro.

SICILIAN TUNA STEAK

START TO FINISH: 45 MINUTES **MAKES:** 4 SERVINGS

450 g/1 lb fresh or frozen tuna steaks, 2.5 cm/1 inch thick
1 small onion, chopped
2 cloves garlic, minced
1 tablespoon extra-virgin olive oil
900 g/2 lb tomatoes, seeded and chopped, or 2 400 g/14 oz cans chopped tomatoes, drained
115 ml/4 fl oz dry white wine
1/4 to 1/2 teaspoon crushed red pepper
40 g/1 1/2 oz pitted ripe olives
2 tablespoons capers, rinsed and drained
2 tablespoons chopped fresh basil or 2 teaspoons dried basil, crushed
1 tablespoon chopped fresh mint or 1 teaspoon dried mint, crushed
1/4 teaspoon sea salt
1/8 teaspoon freshly ground black pepper
1 tablespoon lemon juice

1. Thaw tuna, if frozen. Cut tuna into 4 portions, if necessary. Rinse tuna; pat dry with paper towels. Set aside.

2. In a large frying-pan cook onion and garlic in hot oil over medium heat until onion is tender. Add tomatoes, wine, and crushed red pepper. Bring to boiling; reduce heat. Simmer, uncovered, for 7 minutes. Add olives, capers, and dried basil and mint, if using; cook for 3 minutes more.

3. Sprinkle tuna with sea salt and black pepper. Add tuna to frying-pan on top of tomato mixture. Cover and cook over medium heat for 5 minutes. Uncover and cook for 10 to 15 minutes more or until tuna flakes easily when tested with a fork and is slightly pink in the centre.

4. Transfer tuna pieces to 4 serving plates. Spoon tomato mixture over tuna. Sprinkle with fresh basil and mint, if using. Drizzle with lemon juice.

Nutrition Facts per serving: 233 cal., 6 g total fat (1 g sat. fat), 51 mg chol., 377 mg sodium, 12 g carbo., 3 g fibre, 29 g pro.

MEDITERRANEAN TUNA AND CAPER SALAD

START TO FINISH: 25 MINUTES **MAKES:** 4 SERVINGS

2 tomatoes, chopped
2 tablespoons capers, rinsed and drained
2 tablespoons extra-virgin olive oil
2 tablespoons balsamic vinegar
⅛ teaspoon dried oregano, crushed, or ½ teaspoon chopped fresh oregano
⅛ teaspoon sea salt
   Dash freshly ground black pepper
225 g/8 oz torn mixed salad greens
   2 170 g/6 oz cans tuna (water pack), drained and broken
   into chunks
225 g/8 oz canned chickpeas, rinsed and drained
225 g/8 oz green beans, blanched*
   40 g/1½ oz pitted kalamata olives, quartered
   4 teaspoons extra-virgin olive oil
   4 teaspoons balsamic vinegar

1. In a small bowl combine tomatoes, capers, the 2 tablespoons oil, the 2 tablespoons balsamic vinegar, the oregano, sea salt, and black pepper; set aside.

2. On 4 serving plates, arrange torn salad greens, tuna chunks, chickpeas, green beans, olives, and tomato mixture. Drizzle the 4 teaspoons oil and the 4 teaspoons balsamic vinegar evenly over salads.

Nutrition Facts per serving: 324 cal., 16 g total fat (2 g sat. fat), 36 mg chol., 775 mg sodium, 21 g carbo., 5 g fibre, 25 g pro.

*Note: To blanch the green beans, wash beans; remove ends and strings. Leave beans whole or snap in half. In a covered medium saucepan cook beans in a small amount of boiling lightly salted water for 5 minutes or until crisp-tender. Drain; place in ice water until chilled. Drain well.

ROAST PORK LOIN WITH VEGETABLE RATATOUILLE

PREP: 40 MINUTES **ROAST:** 30 MINUTES **STAND:** 10 MINUTES
OVEN: 220°C/425°F/GAS MARK 7 **MAKES:** 4 SERVINGS

3 cloves garlic, minced
2 teaspoons chopped fresh rosemary or ½ teaspoon dried rosemary, crushed
2 tablespoons extra-virgin olive oil
1 450 to 565 g/1 to 1¼ lb pork tenderloin
2 tablespoons chopped fresh oregano or 2 teaspoons dried oregano, crushed
2 teaspoons finely shredded lemon peel
3 tablespoons lemon juice
450 g/1 lb small courgettes, halved lengthwise
450 g/1 lb yellow pattypan squash, halved lengthwise
1 medium onion, sliced 1 cm/½ inch thick
2 small red peppers, halved and seeded
2 small yellow peppers, halved and seeded
2 medium tomatoes, seeded and chopped
1 tablespoon capers, rinsed and drained
4 large fresh basil leaves, cut into thin strips
Sea salt
Freshly ground black pepper

1. In a small bowl combine 2 cloves of the garlic, the rosemary, and 1 tablespoon of the oil.
Spoon mixture evenly over pork; rub in with your fingers.

2. In the same small bowl combine remaining clove of garlic, remaining 1 tablespoon oil, the
oregano, lemon peel, and lemon juice. Brush over courgettes, pattypan squash, onion, and
peppers.

3. Place a rack in the centre of a large shallow roasting pan. Place tenderloin on rack.
Arrange seasoned vegetables around the edge of the pan. (The vegetables don't need to be
on the rack). Roast in a 220°C/425°F/gas mark 7 oven for 30 to 40 minutes. Remove tenderloin
from roasting pan. Cover with foil and let stand for 10 minutes before slicing. Transfer
vegetables to a very large serving bowl; add tomatoes, capers, and basil. Toss to combine.
Season to taste with sea salt and black pepper. Cover and let stand until pork is ready to
serve.

4. Cut pork into 0.5-cm/¼-inch slices. Serve pork on top of vegetables.

Nutrition Facts per serving: 308 cal., 11 g total fat (2 g sat. fat), 73 mg chol.,
252 mg sodium, 26 g carbo., 7 g fibre, 29 g pro.

Tip: The vegetable ratatouille can also be served as a side dish for roast poultry or it can
be used as a filling in a sandwich with sliced meat.

SPINACH AND LENTIL SALAD WITH TOASTED WALNUTS

START TO FINISH: 30 MINUTES **MAKES:** 4 SERVINGS

225 ml/8 fl oz water
115 g/4 oz brown or French lentils, rinsed and drained
50 g/2 oz chopped red pepper
50 g/2 oz chopped spring onions
3 tablespoons chopped flat-leaf parsley
50 g/2 oz chopped walnuts, toasted
225 g/8 oz torn spinach or mixed salad greens
340 g/12 oz cooked chicken breast, sliced
50 ml/2 fl oz Red Wine Vinaigrette (see recipe, page 152)

1. In a small saucepan combine the water and lentils. Bring to boiling; reduce heat. Cover and simmer for 20 to 25 minutes or until lentils are tender and most of the liquid is absorbed. Drain lentils and place in a medium bowl. Stir in pepper, spring onions, parsley, and walnuts.

2. Divide spinach among 4 serving plates. Top with lentil mixture and chicken. Drizzle with Red Wine Vinaigrette.

Nutrition Facts per serving: 341 cal., 14 g total fat (2 g sat. fat), 72 mg chol., 166 mg sodium, 19 g carbo., 10 g fibre, 36 g pro.

SZECHUAN PRAWNS

PREP: 35 MINUTES **COOK:** 10 MINUTES **MAKES:** 4 SERVINGS

565 g/1¼ lb fresh or frozen medium prawns
  4 teaspoons soy sauce
  4 teaspoons grated fresh ginger or ½ teaspoon ground ginger
  1 tablespoon dry sherry or water
  1 tablespoon Oriental chilli sauce with garlic
  1 teaspoon cornflour
  1 teaspoon toasted sesame oil
⅛ teaspoon sea salt
    Sea salt
    Freshly ground black pepper
1½ teaspoons soy sauce
  ½ teaspoon cornflour
  4 teaspoons olive oil
  3 cloves garlic, minced
115 g/4 oz sliced fresh mushrooms
  1 medium red pepper, cut into 1-cm/½-inch pieces
225 g/8 oz fresh mangetout peas, trimmed
225 g/8 oz shredded Chinese leaves
  40 g/1½ oz dry-roasted peanuts
  2 tablespoons sliced spring onions

1. Thaw prawns, if frozen. Peel and devein prawns. Rinse prawns; pat dry with paper towels. For sauce, in a small bowl combine the 4 teaspoons soy sauce, the ginger, dry sherry or water, Oriental chilli sauce, the 1 teaspoon cornflour, the sesame oil, and the ⅛ teaspoon sea salt. Set aside.

2. Place prawns in a medium bowl; sprinkle lightly with additional sea salt and black pepper. Stir in the 1½ teaspoons soy sauce and the ½ teaspoon cornflour; set aside.

3. In a wok or 30-cm/12-inch frying-pan heat 2 teaspoons of the oil over medium-high heat. Add garlic; stir-fry for 30 seconds. Add mushrooms; stir-fry for 3 minutes. Add pepper; stir-fry for 1 minute. Add mangetout peas; stir-fry for 2 minutes. Remove vegetables from wok.

4. Add remaining 2 teaspoons oil to wok or frying-pan. Add prawn mixture; stir-fry for 2 to 3 minutes or until prawns turn opaque. Stir sauce; add to wok. Cook and stir until boiling; cook and stir for 2 minutes more. Add mushroom mixture and Chinese leaves. Toss to coat.

5. To serve, sprinkle with peanuts and spring onions.

Nutrition Facts per serving: 328 cal., 14 g total fat (2 g sat. fat), 215 mg chol., 714 mg sodium, 16 g carbo., 3 g fibre, 35 g pro.

BAKED EGGS

PREP: 10 MINUTES **BAKE:** 25 MINUTES **OVEN:** 170°C/325°F/GAS MARK 3 **MAKES:** 3 SERVINGS

Non-stick olive oil cooking spray
6 eggs
Chopped fresh chives or desired herb
Sea salt
Freshly ground black pepper
6 tablespoons grated reduced-fat Cheddar or Monterey Jack cheese

1. Coat three 285 g/10 oz baking dishes with non-stick cooking spray. Carefully break 2 eggs into each dish; sprinkle with chives, sea salt, and black pepper. Set dishes in a 33×23×5-cm/13×9×2-inch baking tray; place on an oven rack. Pour hot water around dishes in pan to a depth of 2.5 cm/1 inch.

2. Bake in a 170°C/325°F/gas mark 3 oven for 20 minutes. Sprinkle cheese on top of eggs. Bake for 5 to 10 minutes more or until egg whites are opaque and yolks are firm and cheese is melted.

Nutrition Facts per serving: 188 cal., 13 g total fat (5 g sat. fat), 433 mg chol., 582 mg sodium, 1 g carbo., 0 g fibre, 16 g pro.

GREEK CHICKEN SALAD WITH WHITE BEANS

START TO FINISH: 20 MINUTES **MAKES:** 1 SERVING

1 tablespoon snipped dried tomatoes (not oil-packed)
    Boiling water
85 g/3 oz torn mixed salad greens
85 g/3 oz cooked skinless chicken breast, sliced
50 g/2 oz canned cannellini beans (white kidney beans), rinsed and drained
1 tablespoon crumbled feta cheese
1 tablespoon slivered almonds, toasted
1 tablespoon Red Wine Vinaigrette (see recipe, page 152)

1. Place dried tomatoes in a small bowl. Add enough boiling water to cover; let stand for 5 minutes. Drain well.

2. Meanwhile, arrange salad greens on a serving plate. Top with chicken, cannellini beans, feta cheese, and almonds. Sprinkle with drained tomatoes. Drizzle with Red Wine Vinaigrette.

Nutrition Facts per serving: 326 cal., 15 g total fat (3 g sat. fat), 80 mg chol., 442 mg sodium, 16 g carbo., 6 g fibre, 35g pro.

HALIBUT AND SUMMER VEGETABLES EN PAPILLOTE

PREP: 30 MINUTES **BAKE:** 15 MINUTES **OVEN:** 200°C/400°F/GAS MARK 6 **MAKES:** 4 SERVINGS

4 115 to 150 g/4 to 5 oz fresh or frozen halibut steaks
2 tablespoons extra-virgin olive oil
2 cloves garlic, thinly sliced
  Parchment paper
2 medium tomatoes, sliced 0.5 cm/¼ inch thick
1 medium fennel bulb, cored and sliced
  Sea salt
  Freshly ground black pepper
340 g/12 oz courgettes, bias-sliced 0.5 cm/¼ inch thick
340 g/12 oz yellow pattypan squash, bias-sliced 0.5 cm/¼ inch thick
 40 g/1½ oz pitted kalamata olives, quartered
2 teaspoons finely shredded lemon peel
3 tablespoons lemon juice
2 tablespoons thinly sliced fresh basil or 2 teaspoons dried basil, crushed

1. Thaw halibut, if frozen. Rinse halibut; pat dry with paper towels. In a small saucepan heat oil over low heat. Add garlic; cook for 5 minutes, watching carefully so garlic does not brown. Set aside.

2. Tear four 50×30-cm/20×12-inch pieces of parchment paper; fold each in half crosswise and crease. Open up again. On half of one parchment sheet, arrange one quarter each of the tomato and fennel slices; sprinkle lightly with sea salt and black pepper. Drizzle with some of the oil and garlic mixture. Top with one quarter of the courgettes and yellow pattypan squash; sprinkle again with sea salt and black pepper. Top with one quarter of the olives and one piece of halibut. Sprinkle again with sea salt and black pepper; sprinkle with some of the lemon peel, juice, and basil. To make packet, fold paper over fish and vegetables. Crimp and fold edges to seal; twist corners. Repeat to make 4 packets.

3. Place packets in a shallow baking tray. Bake in a 200°C/400°F/gas mark 6 oven about 15 minutes or until fish flakes easily when tested with a fork. (To test, carefully open the packets and peek.) Serve immediately.

Nutrition Facts per serving: 249 cal., 11 g total fat (1 g sat. fat), 36 mg chol., 648 mg sodium, 13 g carbo., 4 g fibre, 27 g pro.

WAVE 2
MEAL PLANS

For Wave 2, you have two weeks' worth of pre-planned meal plans to follow. Like the Wave 1 meal plans, they suggest three complete meals for you each day, plus two snacks.

Also like Wave 1, these meal plans are optional. You can prepare the suggested meals from the menus, or improvise your own meals following the guidelines for Wave 2 of the Sonoma Diet.

There are two ways that the Wave 2 menus differ from the Wave 1 menus. One is that there are 14 days' worth of recipes instead of 10. Of course, you'll probably need to stay on Wave 2 for more than 14 days before you reach your target weight. You can either keep repeating the 14-day cycle or eventually start choosing new dishes from the additional Wave 2 recipes and/or rearranging the combinations within the Wave 2 guidelines. Using recipes and/or menus from Wave 1 is also an option.

The other major difference is the far greater variety in the Wave 2 meal plans. That's because they take advantage of the ample food choices available to you in this main phase of the Sonoma Diet. You'll never have to worry about boring or unsatisfying meals.

You'll find preparation instructions for the dishes in these meal plans in the Wave 2 meal plan recipe section. Though it's not obligatory, we recommend that you follow these daily meal plans as much as possible for at least the first two weeks of Wave 2. Not only do they take all the guesswork out of adhering to the diet guidelines, they'll also introduce you to new sources of Sonoma-style culinary pleasure and you'll find wine-pairing recommendations (if you choose to drink wine).

DAY ONE

Breakfast: Whole grain cereal and milk

Lunch: Tangy Black Bean Soup (page 202)

Spinach salad with vinaigrette
Try adding chopped sun-dried tomatoes, 1 tablespoon walnuts,
   1 tablespoon mozzarella cheese

115 g / 4 oz fresh berries

Dinner: Latin Spiced Pork Tenderloin (page 203)

Toasted Quinoa Pilaf (page 175)

Roasted Courgettes (page 204)

115 g / 4 oz cantaloupe melon or other Tier 2 fruit

1 glass Pinot Noir or Zinfandel (optional)

Snacks for Men: 2 mozzarella string cheese sticks

2 stalks celery with 2 tablespoons peanut butter

33 almonds

Snacks for Women: 2 stalks celery with 2 tablespoons peanut butter

22 almonds

DAY TWO

Breakfast: 50 g / 2 oz porridge with milk

Lunch: Sonoma Salad with Tomatoes and Feta (page 205)

Fresh fruit of choice

4 whole wheat crackers or 1 small whole wheat pitta bread

Dinner: Prawns with Serrano Chillies (page 206)

Southwestern Grain Medley (page 207)

40 g / 1½ oz baby greens or mixed salad leaves
Try adding 1 tablespoon goat's cheese with balsamic vinaigrette
   or Red Wine Vinaigrette (page 152)

Fruit of choice

1 glass Sauvignon Blanc (optional)

Snacks for Men: 150 g / 5 oz baby carrots

3 Laughing Cow Light cheese spread triangles

33 almonds

Snacks for Women: 150 g / 5 oz baby carrots

1 Laughing Cow Light cheese spread triangle

DAY THREE

Breakfast: 2 eggs

1 slice whole grain toast with 1 tablespoon peanut butter

Lunch: Sonoma Express Wrap (page 127)

170 g / 6 oz Southwestern Grain Medley (from previous evening)

Fresh fruit of choice

Dinner Herbed Pork Tenderloin (page 208)

Spinach with Roasted Garlic Balsamic
Vinaigrette (page 209)

Fresh Fruit of choice

1 glass Zinfandel or Cabernet Sauvignon (optional)

Snacks for Men: 2 tablespoons Yogurt and Cucumber Sauce (page 140)
spread on ½ of a whole wheat pitta bread and
topped with 115 g / 4 oz raw courgette slices

22 almonds

Snacks for Women: 2 tablespoons Yogurt and Cucumber Sauce (page 140)
spread on ½ of a whole wheat pitta bread and
topped with 115 g / 4 oz raw courgette slices

DAY FOUR

Breakfast: 2 slices whole grain bread with 1 tablespoon peanut butter

Lunch: California Chicken Salad (page 210)

1 whole wheat pitta bread

Dinner: Hearty Lentil Soup (page 211)

Fish with Courgette Relish (page 212)

40 g / 1½ oz mixed greens with choice of vinaigrette

1 glass Sauvignon Blanc (optional)

Snacks for Men: 170 g / 6 oz carton plain fat-free yogurt

150 g / 5 oz fresh strawberries

2 Laughing Cow Light cheese spread triangles

150 g / 5 oz raw red pepper strips

22 almonds

Snacks for Women: 170 g / 6 oz carton plain fat-free yogurt

150 g / 5 oz fresh strawberries

2 Laughing Cow Light cheese spread triangles

150 g / 5 oz raw red pepper strips

DAY FIVE

Breakfast: Ranchero Omelette (page 171)

Lunch: Mixed Greens with Turkey and Blue Cheese (page 213)

4 whole wheat crackers

Dinner: Chilli Ginger Beef and Asian Vegetable Medley (page 214)

Fresh fruit of choice

1 glass rosé or sparkling semi-sweet wine (optional)

Snacks for Men: 50 g / 2 oz Hummus (page 149) spread on

1 whole wheat pitta bread and topped with

115 g / 4 oz cucumber slices

2 stalks celery with 2 tablespoons peanut butter

Snacks for Women: 2 tablespoons Hummus (page 149) spread on

1 whole wheat pitta bread and topped with

115 g / 4 oz cucumber slices

DAY SIX

Breakfast: 2 slices whole grain bread with 2 tablespoons peanut butter

Lunch: Greens with Beans and Artichoke Hearts (page 215)

115 g / 4 oz raspberries

Dinner: Grilled Moroccan Pork Tenderloin Kebabs (page 216)

Tunisian Carrot Salad (page 217)

Steamed brown rice

1 glass Zinfandel or Pinot Noir (optional)

Snacks for Men: 115 g / 4 oz broccoli florets

3 Laughing Cow Mini Babybel cheeses

85 g / 3 oz fresh blueberries

150 g / 6 oz carton plain fat-free yogurt

Snacks for Women: 115 g / 4 oz broccoli florets

1 Laughing Cow Mini Babybel cheese

85 g / 3 oz fresh blueberries

150 g / 6 oz carton plain fat-free yogurt

DAY SEVEN

Breakfast:	Whole grain cereal and milk
Lunch:	Chicken and Black Bean Wrap (page 168)
	Fresh fruit of choice
Dinner:	Wild Mushroom and Barley Risotto (page 218)
	Baby Greens with Apples, Walnuts, and Lemon Vinaigrette (page 219)
	1 glass Pinot Noir or Merlot (optional)
Snacks for Men:	33 almonds
	2 celery stalks with 2 tablespoons peanut butter
	1 mozzarella string cheese stick
	150 g / 5 oz baby carrots
Snacks for Women:	11 almonds
	2 celery stalks with 1 tablespoon peanut butter
	1 mozzarella string cheese stick
	150 g / 5 oz baby carrots

DAY EIGHT

Breakfast:	2 eggs
	1 slice whole grain bread with 1 tablespoon peanut butter
Lunch:	Cos Lettuce and Watercress with Vinaigrette (page 220)
	2 whole wheat crackers
Dinner:	Cioppino Seafood en Papillote (page 221)
	50 g / 2 oz cooked whole grain pasta tossed with 1 tablespoon pesto
	70 g / 2½ oz fresh fruit of choice
	1 glass White Zinfandel or Pinot Noir (optional)
Snacks for Men:	115 g / 4 oz low-fat cottage cheese
	115 g / 4 oz grapes
	1 whole wheat pitta bread with 50 g / 2 oz Hummus (page 149) and topped with 150 g / 5 oz raw red pepper strips
	11 almonds
Snacks for Women:	115 g / 4 oz low-fat cottage cheese
	115 g / 4 oz grapes
	½ whole wheat pitta bread with 2 tablespoons Hummus (page 149) and topped with 150 g / 5 oz raw red pepper strips

DAY NINE

Breakfast: 50 g/2 oz porridge with milk
Lunch: Mediterranean White Bean and Spelt Salad (page 222)
70 g/2½ oz fresh fruit of choice
Dinner: Szechuan Beef and Mangetout Stir-Fry (page 223)
Steamed brown rice
70 g/2½ oz fresh fruit of choice
1 glass Zinfandel or sparkling semi-sweet white wine (optional)
Snacks for Men: 3 Laughing Cow Light cheese spread triangles
85 g/3 oz raw courgette slices
33 peanuts
1 hard-boiled egg
Snacks for Women: 1 Laughing Cow Light cheese spread triangle
85 g/3 oz raw courgette slices
22 peanuts

DAY TEN

Breakfast: Florentine Omelette (page 171)
Lunch: Sonoma Express Wrap (page 127)
170 g/6 oz carton plain fat-free yogurt topped with
50 g/2 oz fresh berries and 70 g/2½ oz whole grain cereal
Dinner: Turkey Sausage-Chickpea Soup with Pasta (page 224)
40 g/1½ oz spinach salad with Red Wine Vinaigrette (page 152)
70 g/2½ oz fresh fruit of choice
1 glass Chardonnay (optional)
Snacks for Men: 115 g/4 oz broccoli florets
1 mozzarella string cheese stick
33 almonds
1 slice whole grain bread with 1 tablespoon peanut butter
Snacks for Women: 115 g/4 oz broccoli florets
1 mozzarella string cheese stick
1 slice whole grain bread with 1 tablespoon peanut butter

DAY ELEVEN

Breakfast: Whole grain cereal and milk

Lunch: Tuna Salad Sandwich (page 225)

Fresh fruit of choice

170 g / 5 oz raw pepper strips

Dinner: Chilli-Mint Burgers (page 226)

Green Bean and Tomato Salad (page 227)

70 g / 2½ oz fresh fruit of choice

1 glass rosé or Sauvignon Blanc (optional)

Snacks for Men: 2 celery stalks with 2 tablespoons peanut butter

115 g / 4 oz low-fat cottage cheese

22 almonds

1 hard-boiled egg

Snacks for Women: 2 celery stalks with 2 tablespoons peanut butter

115 g / 4 oz low-fat cottage cheese

11 almonds

DAY TWELVE

Breakfast: 2 slices whole grain bread with 2 tablespoons peanut butter

Lunch: Sonoma Express Wrap (page 127) made with turkey

Try leftover beans and spinach mixture from last evening's salad

70 g / 2½ oz fresh fruit of choice

Dinner: Herb-Roasted Chicken (page 228)

Cauliflower with Parmesan Cheese (page 229)

Wild rice

170 g / 5 oz fresh fruit of choice

1 glass Cabernet Franc, Cabernet Sauvignon, or Merlot (optional)

Snacks for Men: 170 g / 6 oz carton plain fat-free yogurt

50 g / 2 oz strawberries

33 almonds

70 g / 2½ oz baby carrots

2 Laughing Cow Light cheese spread triangles

Snacks for Women: 170 g / 6 oz carton plain fat-free yogurt

50 g / 2 oz strawberries

70 g / 2½ oz baby carrots

1 Laughing Cow Light cheese spread triangle

DAY THIRTEEN

Breakfast: Whole grain cereal and milk

Lunch: Wild Rice Salad with Chicken (page 230)

150 g / 5 oz raw baby carrots and celery with 2 tablespoons Hummus (page 149)

Dinner: Pork Chops with Rosemary (page 231)

Brussels Sprouts with Prosciutto (page 232)

1 slice of rustic whole grain bread

70 g / 2½ oz fresh fruit of choice

1 glass Cabernet Sauvignon, Merlot, or Syrah (optional)

Snacks for Men: 20-cm / 8-inch whole wheat tortilla topped with 25 g / 1 oz grated mozzarella cheese and 50 g / 2 oz broccoli florets. Heat in the microwave oven until cheese is melted; roll up.

33 almonds

Snacks for Women: 20-cm / 8-inch whole wheat tortilla topped with 25 g / 1 oz grated mozzarella cheese and 50 g / 2 oz broccoli florets. Heat in the microwave oven until cheese is melted; roll up.

11 almonds

DAY FOURTEEN

Breakfast: 2 eggs

1 slice whole grain toast with 1 tablespoon peanut butter

Lunch: Greens with Beans and Artichoke Hearts (page 215)

2 whole wheat crackers

Dinner: Greek Pizza (page 233)

150 g / 5 oz raw courgette slices

70 g / 2½ oz fresh fruit of choice

1 glass rosé or Sangiovese (optional)

Snacks for Men: ½ whole wheat pitta bread spread with 2 tablespoons Yogurt and Cucumber Sauce (page 140) and topped with 70 g / 2½ oz roasted red peppers

33 almonds

Snacks for Women: ½ whole wheat pitta bread spread with 2 tablespoons Yogurt and Cucumber Sauce (page 140) and topped with 70 g / 2½ oz roasted red peppers

TANGY BLACK BEAN SOUP

PREP: 35 MINUTES **COOK:** 25 MINUTES **MAKES:** 6 SERVINGS

70 g/2½ oz chopped onion
12 cloves garlic, minced
2 tablespoons extra-virgin olive oil
½ teaspoon ground cumin
2 litres/1¾ pints chicken stock
3 400 g/14 oz cans black beans, rinsed and drained
1 lemon, sliced 1 cm/½ inch thick
50 g/2 oz snipped dried tomatoes (not oil-packed)
1 small fresh jalapeño chilli seeded and finely chopped* (optional)
1 tablespoon chopped fresh oregano or 1 teaspoon dried oregano, crushed
1½ teaspoons sherry vinegar or balsamic vinegar

1. In a 4.5 litre/8-pint heavy casserole cook onion and garlic in hot oil over medium heat until tender, stirring occasionally. Add cumin; cook and stir for 1 minute more. Add stock, beans, lemon slices, tomatoes, chilli (if desired), and dried oregano (if using). Bring to boiling; reduce heat. Simmer, uncovered, for 15 minutes, stirring occasionally.

2. Discard lemon slices. Remove half of the soup mixture to a large heatproof bowl. Use a hand-held blender or potato masher to coarsely purée or mash the mixture in the bowl. Return to casserole. Return to boiling; reduce heat. Cook, uncovered, for 10 minutes more, stirring occasionally.

3. Stir in vinegar and fresh oregano (if using).

Nutrition Facts per serving: 223 cal., 5 g total fat (1 g sat. fat), 0 mg chol., 1,381 mg sodium, 37 g carbo., 12 g fibre, 17 g pro.

*Note: Because chillies contain oils that can burn your skin and eyes, wear rubber or plastic gloves when working with them. If your bare hands do touch the chillies, wash your hands well with soap and water.

To freeze soup: Divide soup among freezer containers; seal, label, and freeze for up to 3 months. Thaw in the refrigerator before heating through.

LATIN SPICED PORK TENDERLOIN

PREP: 10 MINUTES **ROAST:** 25 MINUTES **STAND:** 15 MINUTES
OVEN: 220°C/425°F/GAS MARK 7 **MAKES:** 8 SERVINGS

2 teaspoons chilli powder
1 teaspoon garlic powder
1 teaspoon dried oregano, crushed
¾ teaspoon sea salt
½ teaspoon freshly ground black pepper
½ teaspoon ground cumin
¼ teaspoon cayenne pepper
2 450 g/1 lb pork tenderloins

1. For rub, in a small bowl combine chilli powder, garlic powder, oregano, sea salt, black pepper, cumin, and cayenne pepper. Sprinkle rub evenly over all sides of meat; rub in with your fingers.

2. Place meat on a rack in a shallow roasting pan. Roast in a 220°C/425°F/gas mark 7 oven for 25 to 35 minutes. Cover meat with foil and let stand for 15 minutes before slicing.

Nutrition Facts per serving: 137 cal., 3 g total fat (1 g sat. fat), 73 mg chol., 294 mg sodium, 1 g carbo., 0 g fibre, 24 g pro.

Tip: If desired, serve one tenderloin with the Day 1 menu; reserve the second tenderloin for the Day 2 Sonoma Salad with Tomatoes and Feta.

ROASTED COURGETTES

PREP: 15 MINUTES **ROAST:** 20 MINUTES **OVEN:** 220°C/425°F/GAS MARK 7 **MAKES:** 4 SERVINGS

2 cloves garlic, minced
1 tablespoon extra-virgin olive oil
1 tablespoon chopped fresh rosemary or ½ teaspoon dried rosemary, crushed
½ teaspoon freshly ground black pepper
¼ teaspoon sea salt
675 g/1½ lb courgettes and/or yellow pattypan squash, sliced 1 cm/½ inch thick

1. In a small saucepan cook garlic in hot oil over medium heat for 30 seconds. Stir in rosemary, black pepper, and sea salt.

2. Place courgettes and/or pattypan squash in a 33×23×5-cm/13×9×2-inch baking pan; add oil mixture. Toss to coat. Roast, uncovered, in a 220°C/425°/gas mark 7 oven about 20 minutes or until crisp-tender, stirring once.

Nutrition Facts per serving: 61 cal., 4 g total fat (1 g sat. fat), 0 mg chol., 138 mg sodium, 6 g carbo., 2 g fibre, 2 g pro.

SONOMA SALAD WITH TOMATOES AND FETA

START TO FINISH: 20 MINUTES **MAKES:** 4 SERVINGS

340 g/12 oz torn mixed salad greens
340 g/12 oz cooked skinless chicken or turkey breast, lean beef, or pork, sliced
150 g/5 oz cherry tomatoes, halved
 50 g/2 oz sliced, halved cucumber
 3 tablespoons small fresh basil leaves
 1 recipe Red Wine Vinaigrette (see recipe, page 152)
   Sea salt
   Freshly ground black pepper
 25 g/1 oz crumbled feta or goat's cheese
 1 tablespoon pino nuts, toasted

1. In a very large bowl combine greens, meat, tomatoes, cucumber, and basil. Drizzle with Red Wine Vinaigrette. Toss to coat. Season to taste with sea salt and black pepper. Top with feta or goat's cheese and pine nuts. Serve immediately.

Nutrition Facts per serving: 267 cal., 13 g total fat (3 g sat. fat), 80 mg chol., 318 mg sodium, 6 g carbo., 2 g fibre, 30 g pro.

PRAWNS WITH SERRANO CHILLIES

START TO FINISH: 25 MINUTES **MAKES:** 4 SERVINGS

450 g/1 lb fresh or frozen peeled and deveined medium prawns
2 tablespoons extra-virgin olive oil
40 g/1½ oz chopped shallots
3 cloves garlic, minced
40 g/1½ oz chopped red pepper
2 to 3 fresh serrano or jalapeño chillies, seeded and finely chopped*
1 tablespoon lemon juice
1 tablespoon chopped fresh coriander

1. Thaw prawns, if frozen. Rinse prawns; pat dry with paper towels. Set aside.

2. In a large frying-pan heat oil over medium-high heat. Add shallots and garlic; stir-fry for 1 minute. Add peppers and chillies. Stir-fry for 1 minute more. Add prawns; stir-fry for 2 to 3 minutes or until prawns are opaque. Drizzle with lemon juice. Sprinkle with coriander.

Nutrition Facts per serving: 195 cal., 9 g total fat (1 g sat. fat), 172 mg chol., 171 mg sodium, 5 g carbo., 0 g fibre, 24 g pro.

*Note: Because chillies contain oils that can burn your skin and eyes, wear rubber or plastic gloves when working with them. If your bare hands do touch the chillies, wash your hands well with soap and water.

SOUTHWESTERN GRAIN MEDLEY

START TO FINISH: 30 MINUTES **MAKES:** 4 SERVINGS

- 115 g/4 oz fresh or frozen sweetcorn kernels
- 1 teaspoon extra-virgin olive oil
- 150 g/5 oz cooked quinoa*
- 70 g/2½ oz cooked brown or wild rice
- 115 g/4 oz canned black beans, rinsed and drained
- 70 g/2½ oz finely chopped red pepper
- 70 g/2½ oz finely chopped green pepper
- 50 g/2 oz finely chopped, seeded cucumber
- 2 tablespoons thinly sliced spring onion
- 2 tablespoons lime juice
- 1 tablespoon extra-virgin olive oil
- 1½ teaspoons finely chopped fresh jalapeño or serrano chilli**
- 1½ teaspoons chopped fresh coriander
-     Sea salt
-     Freshly ground black pepper

1. Thaw sweetcorn, if frozen. Heat a large non-stick frying-pan over medium-high heat. Add the sweetcorn and the 1 teaspoon oil. Cook and stir about 5 minutes or until browned and toasted. Transfer to a large bowl. Add the quinoa, rice, black beans, peppers, cucumber, spring onion, lime juice, the 1 tablespoon oil, chilli, and coriander. Mix well; season to taste with sea salt and black pepper.

Nutrition Facts per serving: 174 cal., 6 g total fat (1 g sat. fat), 0 mg chol., 154 mg sodium, 28 g carbo., 4 g fibre, 6 g pro.

*Note: Look for quinoa at a health food shop or in the grains section of a large supermarket. To cook quinoa, in a small saucepan add 50 g/2 oz to 115 ml/4 fl oz boiling water. Cover and simmer about 20 minutes or until quinoa is tender and water is absorbed.

**Note: Because chillies contain oils that can burn your skin and eyes, wear rubber or plastic gloves when working with them. If your bare hands do touch the chillies, wash your hands well with soap and water.

HERBED PORK TENDERLOIN

PREP: 15 MINUTES **MARINATE:** 2 TO 4 HOURS **ROAST:** 25 MINUTES
STAND: 15 MINUTES **OVEN:** 220°C/425°F/GAS MARK 7
MAKES: 8 SERVINGS

2 340 g/12 oz pork tenderloins
Sea salt (optional)
Freshly ground black pepper (optional)
2 tablespoons balsamic vinegar
2 tablespoons dry sherry
1 tablespoon cracked black pepper
1 tablespoon extra-virgin olive oil
1 tablespoon soy sauce
2 8-cm/3-inch sprigs fresh rosemary
2 8-cm/3-inch sprigs fresh marjoram
2 8-cm/3-inch sprigs fresh thyme
2 cloves garlic, minced
2 tablespoons extra-virgin olive oil

1. If desired, season meat with sea salt and ground black pepper. Place meat in a large self-sealing plastic bag set in a shallow dish. Set aside.

2. For marinade, in a small bowl stir together vinegar, sherry, the 1 tablespoon cracked black pepper, the 1 tablespoon oil, soy sauce, rosemary, marjoram, thyme, and garlic. Pour over meat. Seal bag; turn to coat meat. Marinate in the refrigerator for 2 to 4 hours, turning bag occasionally.

3. Drain meat, reserving marinade. In a large frying-pan heat the 2 tablespoons oil. Brown meat quickly on all sides in hot oil (about 5 minutes).

4. Place meat in a shallow roasting pan. Pour marinade over meat. Roast, uncovered, in a 220°C/425°F/gas mark 7 oven for 15 minutes. Spoon pan juices over meat. Roast for 10 to 15 minutes more, then cover roast with foil and let stand for 15 minutes. Transfer meat to a serving platter, reserving pan juices. Strain juices and pour over meat.

Nutrition Facts per serving: 159 cal., 8 g total fat (2 g sat. fat), 55 mg chol., 155 mg sodium, 2 g carbo., 0 g fibre, 18 g pro.

Spinach with Roasted Garlic Balsamic Vinaigrette

PREP: 30 MINUTES **ROAST:** 30 MINUTES (GARLIC)
OVEN: 180°C/350°F/GAS MARK 4 **MAKES:** 4 SERVINGS

2 tablespoons balsamic vinegar
1 teaspoon lemon juice
1 tablespoon finely chopped shallot
1 teaspoon Roasted Garlic Purée
2 tablespoons extra-virgin olive oil
⅛ teaspoon sea salt
   Dash freshly ground black pepper
115 g/4 oz torn frisée or endive
115 g/4 oz whole fresh baby spinach leaves
50 g/2 oz fresh mushrooms, sliced
70 g/2½ oz cup cherry tomatoes, halved
2 tablespoons pine nuts, toasted
2 tablespoons finely grated Parmesan cheese

1. For vinaigrette, in a small bowl combine vinegar, lemon juice, and shallot. Let stand for 5 minutes. Whisk in the Roasted Garlic Purée; whisk in oil, sea salt, and black pepper until combined.

2. In a large bowl combine frisée or endive, spinach, mushrooms, tomatoes, and pine nuts. Drizzle with the vinaigrette; toss to coat. Sprinkle with cheese. Serve immediately.

Roasted Garlic Purée: Slice the top off a garlic bulb to expose the cloves. Rub the bulb with extra-virgin olive oil, then place cut side down in a small baking dish. Cover. Roast in a 200°C/400°F/gas mark 6 oven for 30 to 45 minutes or until soft. Cool. Remove the outer papery covering. Separate into cloves; squeeze out the roasted garlic. Mash lightly with a fork. Use roasted garlic in soups, vegetable purées, sauces, vinaigrettes, or as a spread for crackers.

Nutrition Facts per serving: 123 cal., 10 g total fat (2 g sat. fat), 2 mg chol., 131 mg sodium, 6 g carbo., 2 g fibre, 4 g pro.

Tip: For a main dish, serve the salad with 340 g/12 oz cooked lean pork, skinless chicken breast, or lean beef.

CALIFORNIA CHICKEN SALAD

START TO FINISH: 35 MINUTES **MAKES:** 6 SERVINGS

450 g/1 lb cubed cooked chicken breast
2 Granny Smith apples, cored and chopped
115 g/4 oz chopped celery
70 g/2½ oz chopped spring onions
2 tablespoons chopped fresh flat-leaf parsley
50 ml/2 fl oz low-fat soured cream
50 ml/2 fl oz red wine vinegar
3 tablespoons mayonnaise or salad dressing
½ teaspoon sea salt
¼ teaspoon freshly ground black pepper
25 g/1 oz chopped walnuts, toasted
225 g/8 oz torn mixed salad greens

1. In a large bowl combine chicken, apples, celery, spring onions, and parsley. Stir in soured cream, red wine vinegar, mayonnaise, sea salt, and black pepper. Stir walnuts into chicken mixture. Divide greens among 6 serving plates; top with chicken mixture.

Nutrition Facts per serving: 258 cal., 12 g total fat (2 g sat. fat), 70 mg chol., 288 mg sodium, 11 g carbo., 3 g fibre, 26 g pro.

HEARTY LENTIL SOUP

PREP: 30 MINUTES **COOK:** 30 MINUTES **MAKES:** 6 SERVINGS

1 medium onion, chopped
1 medium carrot, chopped
3 cloves garlic, minced
2 tablespoons extra-virgin olive oil
2 litres/1¾ pints chicken stock
340 g/12 oz brown or French lentils, rinsed and drained
1 medium tomato, seeded and chopped
3 tablespoons chopped fresh flat-leaf parsley
1 tablespoon lemon juice
½ teaspoon cumin seeds, toasted and ground,*
    or ½ teaspoon ground cumin
½ teaspoon fennel seeds, toasted and ground,*
    or ½ teaspoon fennel seeds, finely crushed
    Sea salt (optional)
    Freshly ground black pepper (optional)

1. In a 6.6-litre/12-pint heavy casserole cook onion, carrot, and garlic in hot oil about 10 minutes or until tender.

2. Add stock and lentils to onion mixture. Bring to boiling; reduce heat. Cover and simmer about 30 minutes or until lentils are tender.

3. Stir in tomato, parsley, lemon juice, cumin, and ground fennel seeds. If desired, season to taste with sea salt and black pepper. Ladle into bowls.

Nutrition Facts per serving: 240 cal., 5 g total fat (1 g sat. fat), 0 mg chol., 775 mg sodium, 33 g carbo., 16 g fibre, 17 g pro.

*Note: To toast seeds, heat a small frying-pan over medium heat. Add seeds. Cook about 2 minutes or until toasted and aromatic, shaking pan frequently. Place toasted seeds in a spice grinder and process until finely ground.

FISH WITH COURGETTE RELISH

PREP: 15 MINUTES **BAKE:** 4 MINUTES PER 1-CM ½-INCH THICKNESS
OVEN: 230°C/450°F/GAS MARK 8 **MAKES:** 4 SERVINGS

450 g/1 lb fresh or frozen skinless tilapia fillets
150 g/5 oz chopped courgette or cucumber
70 g/2½ oz chopped red pepper
40 g/1½ oz finely chopped onion
1 small fresh jalapeño chilli, seeded and finely chopped*
1 tablespoon white wine vinegar
1 tablespoon extra-virgin olive oil
½ teaspoon sea salt
¼ teaspoon ground cumin
¼ teaspoon freshly ground black pepper
1 tablespoon extra-virgin olive oil
Fresh tomato wedges (optional)

1. Thaw fish, if frozen. Rinse fish; pat dry with paper towels. Cut into 4 serving-size pieces, if necessary. Measure thickness of fish. Set aside. For the courgette relish, in a medium bowl combine courgettes, pepper, onion, chilli, white wine vinegar, 1 tablespoon olive oil, and ¼ teaspoon of the sea salt. Set aside.

2. In a small bowl combine remaining ¼ teaspoon sea salt, the cumin, and black pepper. Arrange fish in a single layer in a 38×25×2.5-cm/15×10×1-inch baking pan, turning under thin edges. Sprinkle cumin mixture evenly over fish. Drizzle with 1 tablespoon oil.

3. Bake in a 230°C/450°F/gas mark 8 oven for 4 to 6 minutes per 1-cm/½-inch thickness of fish or until fish flakes easily when tested with a fork.

4. Serve fish with courgette relish and, if desired, tomato wedges.

Nutrition Facts per serving: 170 cal., 8 g total fat (1 g sat. fat), 48 mg chol., 357 mg sodium, 4 g carbo., 1 g fibre, 21 g pro.

*Note: Because chillies contain oils that can burn your skin and eyes, wear rubber or plastic gloves when working with them. If your bare hands do touch the chillies, wash your hands well with soap and water.

MIXED GREENS WITH TURKEY AND BLUE CHEESE

START TO FINISH: 20 MINUTES **MAKES:** 4 SERVINGS

170 g/6 oz torn mixed salad greens
340 g/12 oz cooked skinless chicken or turkey breast, sliced
  2 pears, cored and sliced
  25 g/1 oz walnut pieces, toasted
  25 g/1 oz crumbled blue cheese
  1 recipe Mustard-Red Wine Vinaigrette

1. In a large bowl combine greens, chicken, pears, walnuts, and blue cheese. Add the Mustard-Red Wine Vinaigrette; toss to coat. Serve immediately.

Mustard-Red Wine Vinaigrette: In a small bowl combine 50 ml/2 fl oz red wine vinegar, 2 tablespoons finely chopped shallots, and 1 clove garlic, minced. Let stand for 5 minutes. Whisk in 3 tablespoons extra-virgin olive oil, 1½ teaspoons Dijon-style mustard, ¼ teaspoon sea salt, and ¼ teaspoon freshly ground black pepper.

Nutrition Facts per serving: 378 cal., 21 g total fat (4 g sat. fat), 79 mg chol., 362 mg sodium, 18 g carbo., 5 g fibre, 31 g pro.

CHILLI GINGER BEEF AND ASIAN VEGETABLE MEDLEY

PREP: 1 HOUR **MARINATE:** 30 MINUTES TO 1 HOUR
GRILL: 17 MINUTES **MAKES:** 6 SERVINGS

1 565 g/1¼ lb beef steak
1 recipe Chilli-Herb Dressing
225 g/8 oz fresh sugar snap peas or mangetout peas, trimmed
115 g/4 oz shredded Chinese leaves
225 g/8 oz carrots, thinly sliced
150 g/5 oz shelled fresh or frozen sweet soya beans (edamame), thawed
150 g/5 oz radishes, thinly sliced
150 g/5 oz green and/or red pepper strips
3 tablespoons chopped fresh coriander
40 g/1½ oz chopped spring onions
2 tablespoons chopped dry roasted peanuts

1. Trim fat from steak. Score both sides of steak in a diamond pattern by making shallow cuts at 2.5-cm/1-inch intervals. Place steak in a self-sealing plastic bag set in a shallow dish. Pour half of the Chilli-Herb Dressing over the steak; reserve remaining dressing for salad. Seal bag; turn bag to coat steak. Marinate in the refrigerator for 30 minutes to 1 hour, turning bag once.

2. Meanwhile, for salad, in a covered medium saucepan cook sugar snap peas in a small amount of boiling water for 1 minute; drain. Submerse in ice water to cool quickly; drain. In a large bowl combine the sugar snap peas, Chinese leaves, carrots, soya beans, radishes, pepper strips, coriander, and the spring onions. Add remaining Chilli-Herb Dressing; toss to coat. Cover and chill until serving time.

3. Drain steak, discarding marinade. Place steak on the rack of a grill or barbecue and grill for 17 to 21 minutes or until desired doneness, turning once halfway through grilling. To serve, thinly slice steak across the grain.

4. Serve steak slices with the chilled salad. Sprinkle with peanuts.

Chilli-Herb Dressing: In a screw-top jar combine 85 ml/3 fl oz soy sauce; 85 ml/3 fl oz rice vinegar; 2 tablespoons grated fresh ginger; 2 fresh serrano chillies, seeded and finely chopped*; 2 tablespoons chopped fresh basil or 2 teaspoons dried basil, crushed; 2 tablespoons chopped fresh mint or 2 teaspoons dried mint, crushed; 2 tablespoons chopped fresh coriander; 6 cloves garlic, minced; and 1 tablespoon toasted sesame oil. Cover and shake well.

Nutrition Facts per serving: 313 cal., 13 g total fat (4 g sat. fat), 38 mg chol., 770 mg sodium, 18 g carbo., 6 g dietary fibre, 30 g protein.

*Note: Because chillies contain oils that can burn your skin and eyes, wear rubber or plastic gloves when working with them. If your bare hands do touch the chillies, wash your hands well with soap and water.

GREENS WITH BEANS AND ARTICHOKE HEARTS

START TO FINISH: 25 MINUTES **MAKES:** 4 SERVINGS

170 g/6 oz torn mixed baby salad greens
1 400 g/14 oz can artichoke hearts, drained and sliced
340 g/12 oz cooked skinless chicken or turkey breast, sliced
225 g/8 oz canned white beans, rinsed and drained
2 tablespoons finely chopped red onion
1 recipe Red Wine Vinaigrette (see recipe, page 152)
25 g/1 oz crumbled goat's cheese
2 tablespoons pine nuts, toasted
1 tablespoon chopped fresh flat-leaf parsley or basil

1. In a large bowl combine baby greens, artichokes, chicken, beans, and red onion. Drizzle with Red Wine Vinaigrette; toss to coat. Top with goat's cheese, pine nuts, and parsley or basil. Serve immediately.

Nutrition Facts per serving: 356 cal., 15 g total fat (4 g sat. fat), 78 mg chol., 553 mg sodium, 20 g carbo., 7 g fibre, 36 g pro.

GRILLED MOROCCAN PORK TENDERLOIN KEBABS

PREP: 35 MINUTES **MARINATE:** 1 TO 2 HOURS **GRILL:** 10 MINUTES
MAKES: 4 SERVINGS

  2 tablespoons chopped fresh flat-leaf parsley
  2 tablespoons lemon juice
  1 tablespoon extra-virgin olive oil
  8 cloves garlic, minced
  1 tablespoon chopped fresh oregano or 1 teaspoon dried oregano, crushed
  1½ teaspoons coriander seeds, ground, or 1 teaspoon ground coriander
  1 teaspoon paprika
  1 teaspoon grated fresh ginger
  ½ teaspoon freshly ground black pepper
  ¼ teaspoon sea salt
  ¼ teaspoon cayenne pepper or crushed red pepper
  ¼ teaspoon ground turmeric
  1 450 g/1 lb pork tenderloin, cut into 2.5-cm/1-inch cubes*
  225 g/8 oz seedless green grapes

1. For marinade, in a large bowl stir together parsley, lemon juice, oil, garlic, oregano, coriander, paprika, ginger, black pepper, sea salt, cayenne pepper, and turmeric until combined. Add pork cubes and grapes. Stir gently until pork and grapes are coated. Cover and marinate in the refrigerator for 1 to 2 hours.

2. On eight 30-cm/12-inch skewers,** alternately thread pork and grapes, leaving a 0.5 cm/¼-inch space between pieces. Place kebabs on the rack of a grill or barbecue and grill for 10 to 12 minutes or until pork is just slightly pink in centre, turning occasionally to brown evenly.

Nutrition Facts per serving: 211 cal., 7 g total fat (2 g sat. fat), 73 mg chol., 170 mg sodium, 12 g carbo., 1 g fibre, 25 g pro.

*Tip: You may substitute 450 g/1 lb skinless, boneless chicken breast halves for the pork.

**Note: If using wooden skewers, soak in enough water to cover for at least 1 hour before using.

Tunisian Carrot Salad

PREP: 20 MINUTES **COOK:** 5 MINUTES **STAND:** 30 MINUTES
MAKES: 4 SERVINGS

450 g/1 lb carrots, sliced 0.5 to 1 cm/¼ to ½ inch thick
50 ml/2 fl oz Harissa Sauce (see recipe, page 142)
1 clove garlic, minced
40 g/1½ oz pitted kalamata olives, coarsely chopped
25 g/1 oz crumbled feta cheese
4 lemon wedges

1. In a covered large saucepan cook carrots in a small amount of boiling water for 5 minutes. Drain; rinse with cold water to cool quickly. Drain well. Place carrots in a medium bowl. Add Harissa Sauce and garlic; toss to combine. Cover and let stand at room temperature for 30 minutes to develop flavours; stir occasionally.

2. Sprinkle servings with olives and feta cheese. Serve with lemon wedges.

Nutrition Facts per serving: 136 cal., 8 g total fat (2 g sat. fat), 8 mg chol., 340 mg sodium, 18 g carbo., 6 g fibre, 3 g pro.

WILD MUSHROOM AND BARLEY RISOTTO

PREP: 35 MINUTES **COOK:** 1 HOUR **MAKES:** 5 SERVINGS

40 g/1½ oz fresh chanterelle, stemmed oyster, and/or stemmed shiitake mushrooms, sliced
1 large shallot, finely chopped
1 clove garlic, minced
1 tablespoon extra-virgin olive oil
85 ml/3 fl oz dry white wine
850 ml/1½ pints chicken stock
90 g/3½ oz regular barley
Chopped fresh flat-leaf parsley

1. In a large frying-pan cook mushrooms, shallot, and garlic in hot oil over medium heat for 5 to 10 minutes or until mushrooms are tender and lightly browned. Add wine. Bring to boiling; reduce heat. Simmer, uncovered, about 5 minutes or until liquid is nearly evaporated.

2. Meanwhile, in a medium saucepan bring chicken stock to boiling; reduce heat. Keep hot over very low heat.

3. Add barley to mushroom mixture; stir to coat. Add 225 ml/8 fl oz of the hot stock to the barley mixture. Cook over medium heat until liquid is absorbed, stirring occasionally. (This should take about 15 minutes. If the liquid absorbs too quickly, reduce the heat.) Repeat with 450 ml/¾ pint more of the hot stock, adding half the stock at a time and cooking until all the liquid is absorbed before adding more, stirring occasionally. (This should take about 30 minutes.)

4. Stir in the remaining hot stock. Cook until the barley is slightly creamy and just tender. (This should take about 15 minutes. Increase the heat slightly if the mixture is too wet.) Sprinkle with parsley.

Nutrition Facts per serving: 145 cal., 3 g total fat (0 g sat. fat), 0 mg chol., 366 mg sodium, 23 g carbo., 4 g fibre, 5 g pro.

BABY GREENS WITH APPLES, WALNUTS, AND LEMON VINAIGRETTE

START TO FINISH: 25 MINUTES **MAKES:** 4 SERVINGS

2 tablespoons lemon juice
2 tablespoons finely chopped shallots
1 tablespoon white wine vinegar
2 tablespoons extra-virgin olive oil
¼ teaspoon sea salt
⅛ teaspoon freshly ground black pepper
225 g/8 oz torn mixed salad greens
3 Granny Smith apples, cored and cut into bite-size strips
40 g/1½ oz fresh flat-leaf parsley leaves
70 g/2½ oz sliced cucumber
25 g/1 oz walnut pieces, toasted
340 g/12 oz cooked skinless chicken breast halves, sliced, or
    8 hard-boiled eggs, peeled and halved

1. For vinaigrette, in a small bowl combine lemon juice, shallots, and vinegar. Let stand for 5 minutes. Whisk in oil, sea salt, and black pepper until well mixed.

2. In a large bowl combine the greens, apples, parsley leaves, cucumber, and walnuts. Add vinaigrette; toss lightly to coat. Divide among 4 serving plates. Top with chicken or eggs. Serve immediately.

Nutrition Facts per serving: 327 cal., 15 g total fat (2 g sat. fat), 72 mg chol., 203 mg sodium, 20 g carbo., 5 g fibre, 29 g pro.

Tip: For extra flavour, top each serving with a tablespoon of goat's cheese.

COS LETTUCE AND WATERCRESS WITH VINAIGRETTE

START TO FINISH: 30 MINUTES **MAKES:** 4 SERVINGS

50 ml/2 fl oz red wine vinegar
2 tablespoons finely chopped shallots
1 clove garlic, minced
1½ teaspoons Dijon-style mustard
3 tablespoons extra-virgin olive oil
¼ teaspoon sea salt
⅛ teaspoon freshly ground black pepper
2 cos lettuces, thinly sliced crosswise
115 g/4 oz watercress or fresh spinach, large stems removed
2 medium carrots, halved lengthwise and thinly sliced
1 medium red pepper, seeded and chopped
2 spring onions, thinly sliced
25 g/1 oz sliced almonds, toasted
340 g/12 oz cooked skinless chicken breast halves, sliced, or 8 hard-boiled
    eggs, peeled and sliced
1 tablespoon finely grated Parmesan cheese

1. For the vinaigrette, in a small bowl combine vinegar, shallots, and garlic. Let stand for 5 minutes. Whisk in mustard. Add oil in a thin, steady stream, whisking constantly until combined. Stir in sea salt and black pepper.

2. In a large bowl combine lettuce, watercress or spinach, carrots, pepper, spring onions, and almonds. Add the vinaigrette; toss to coat. Divide among 4 serving plates. Top servings with chicken or egg slices and sprinkle with cheese. Serve immediately.

Nutrition Facts per serving: 334 cal., 18 g total fat (3 g sat. fat), 73 mg chol., 294 mg sodium, 13 g carbo., 5 g fibre, 32 g pro.

CIOPPINO SEAFOOD EN PAPILLOTE

PREP: 35 MINUTES **BAKE:** 12 MINUTES **OVEN:** 200°C/400°F/GAS MARK 6 **MAKES:** 4 SERVINGS

> **225 g/8 oz fresh or frozen large prawns in shells***
> **225 g/8 oz fresh or frozen sea scallops or 275 g/10 oz fresh or frozen halibut steaks***
> **Parchment paper or foil**
> **2 medium tomatoes, seeded and chopped**
> **1 tablespoon lemon juice**
> **1½ teaspoons chopped fresh basil or ½ teaspoon dried basil, crushed**
> **1½ teaspoons chopped fresh thyme or ½ teaspoon dried thyme, crushed**
> **1 teaspoon extra-virgin olive oil**
> **1 clove garlic, minced**
> **¼ teaspoon sea salt**
> **Pinch saffron, crushed, or ¼ teaspoon ground turmeric**
> **1 small courgette, halved lengthwise and sliced 0.5 cm/¼ inch thick**
> **4 spring onions, cut into 2.5-cm/1-inch pieces**

1. Thaw prawns and scallops or halibut, if frozen. Peel and devein prawns. Halve any large scallops or skin, bone, and cut halibut into 2.5-cm/1-inch pieces. Set aside.

2. Cut four 30-cm/12-inch squares of parchment paper or foil. Fold each square in half to form a triangle. Open each triangle to lie flat.

3. In a large bowl combine tomatoes, lemon juice, basil, thyme, oil, garlic, sea salt, and saffron. Add prawns, scallops, courgettes, and spring onions; toss to coat. Divide mixture among parchment or foil triangles, spooning it onto centre of one side of each triangle. Fold paper or foil over mixture. To seal packets, fold each of the open sides over 1 cm/½ inch, then fold over again 1 cm/½ inch.

4. Place packets on a very large baking sheet. Bake in a 200°C/400°F/gas mark 6 oven for 12 to 15 minutes or until prawns and scallops are opaque or halibut flakes easily when tested with a fork. (To test, carefully open the packets and peek.)

Nutrition Facts per serving: 141 cal., 3 g total fat (0 g sat. fat), 105 mg chol., 305 mg sodium, 6 g carbo., 1 g fibre, 22 g pro.

*Note: If desired, use 450 g/1 lb large prawns in shells and omit the scallops or halibut.

MEDITERRANEAN WHITE BEAN AND SPELT SALAD

PREP: 30 MINUTES **COOK:** 45 MINUTES **MAKES:** 6 SERVINGS

700 ml/1¼ pints water
200 g/7 oz whole spelt or wheat berries
450 g/1 lb green beans, trimmed and cut into 5-cm/2-inch pieces
   1 400 g/14 oz can haricot or cannellini beans, rinsed and drained
115 g/4 oz cherry tomatoes, halved
   40 g/1½ oz pitted kalamata olives, quartered
   85 ml/3 fl oz Pesto Vinaigrette (see recipe, page 155)
   2 170 g/6 oz cans tuna (water pack), drained and broken into chunks;
      340 g/12 oz mozzarella cheese, cut up; or 12 hard-boiled eggs, peeled and
      halved

1. In a medium saucepan combine the water and spelt. Bring to boiling; reduce heat. Cover and simmer for 45 to 60 minutes or until tender. (Or soak grain in water in the refrigerator for 6 to 24 hours. Do not drain. Bring to boiling; reduce heat. Cover and simmer for 30 minutes.) Drain. Run cold water over cooked grain until completely cooled; drain.

2. Meanwhile, in a covered medium saucepan cook green beans in a small amount of boiling salted water for 5 minutes or until crisp-tender. Drain. Place in a bowl of ice water to stop cooking and chill thoroughly; drain.

3. In a large bowl combine cooked grain, green beans, haricot or cannellini beans, tomatoes, and olives. Add Pesto Vinaigrette; toss to coat. Serve immediately with tuna, cheese, or eggs.

Nutrition Facts per serving: 387 cal., 12 g total fat (2 g sat. fat), 24 mg chol., 356 mg sodium, 46 g carbo., 10 g fibre, 25 g pro.

SZECHUAN BEEF AND MANGETOUT STIR-FRY

PREP: 20 MINUTES **STAND:** 15 MINUTES **COOK:** 10 MINUTES
MAKES: 4 SERVINGS

450 g/1 lb beef sirloin steak
1 tablespoon soy sauce
1 teaspoon cornflour
3 tablespoons soy sauce
2 tablespoons dry sherry or water
2 tablespoons Oriental chilli sauce with garlic
2 tablespoons water
1 tablespoon cornflour
1 tablespoon toasted sesame oil
1 tablespoon olive oil
3 cloves garlic, minced
2 tablespoons minced fresh ginger
225 g/8 oz mushrooms, quartered
3 carrots, halved lengthwise and thinly sliced
2 medium red peppers, cut into thin bite-size strips
225 g/8 oz mangetout peas, trimmed and halved crosswise
1 spring onion, thinly sliced

1. Trim fat from beef; cut beef into thin bite-size strips. Place beef in a medium bowl. Add the 1 tablespoon soy sauce and the 1 teaspoon cornflour; stir to combine. Cover and let stand for 15 minutes. Meanwhile, for sauce, stir together the 3 tablespoons soy sauce, the sherry, chilli sauce, the water, the 1 tablespoon cornflour, and sesame oil; set aside.

2. In a wok or very large frying-pan heat olive oil over medium-high heat. Add garlic and ginger; stir-fry for 30 seconds. Add mushrooms; stir-fry for 1 minute. Add carrots; stir-fry for 2 minutes. Add peppers and mangetout peas; stir-fry for 2 minutes. Remove vegetables from wok or frying-pan.

3. Add beef mixture to wok or frying-pan; stir-fry for 2 to 3 minutes or until desired doneness. Stir sauce; add to wok or frying-pan. Cook and stir until thickened and bubbly. Cook and stir for 2 minutes more. Return vegetables to wok or frying-pan. Stir to coat with sauce. Cook and stir until heated through.

4. Sprinkle with spring onion to serve.

Nutrition Facts per serving: 328 cal., 13 g total fat (2 g sat. fat), 69 mg chol., 775 mg sodium, 21 g carbo., 5 g fibre, 30 g pro.

TURKEY SAUSAGE-CHICKPEA SOUP WITH PASTA

PREP: 15 MINUTES **COOK:** 9 MINUTES **MAKES:** 6 SERVINGS

170 g/6 oz uncooked Italian turkey sausage links, casings removed
150 g/5 oz chopped onion
3 cloves garlic, minced
2 tablespoons chopped fresh sage or 2 teaspoons dried sage, crushed
2 tablespoons chopped fresh rosemary or 1½ teaspoons dried rosemary, crushed
1.2 litres/2 pints chicken stock
1 400 g/14 oz can chickpeas, rinsed and drained
170 ml/6 fl oz water
85 g/3 oz tomato purée
85 g/3 oz whole grain pasta
Freshly ground black pepper

1. In a large saucepan* cook sausage, onion, and garlic over medium heat until meat is browned and onion is tender. Stir in sage and rosemary; cook over low heat for 1 minute (do not brown herbs).

2. Stir in stock, chickpeas, water, and tomato purée. Bring to boiling. Stir in uncooked pasta. Simmer, uncovered, for 9 to 11 minutes or until pasta is tender. Season to taste with black pepper.

Nutrition Facts per serving: 213 cal., 4 g total fat (1 g sat. fat), 20 mg chol., 1,331 mg sodium, 31 g carbo., 5 g fibre, 13 g pro.

*Note: If using a regular saucepan, you may need to add 1 to 2 teaspoons extra-virgin olive oil to prevent sticking. If using a non-stick pan, no oil is needed.

TUNA SALAD SANDWICH

START TO FINISH: 10 MINUTES **MAKES:** 1 SERVING

1 85 g/3 oz can tuna (water pack), drained and flaked*
1 tablespoon mayonnaise or salad dressing
1 teaspoon pickle relish
1 tablespoon finely chopped celery
1 tablespoon finely chopped red onion
1 teaspoon Dijon-style mustard
½ teaspoon lemon juice
  Dash sea salt
  Dash garlic powder
  Dash Worcestershire sauce
  Dash freshly ground black pepper
2 slices whole grain bread
1 leaf cos lettuce

1. In a small bowl stir together tuna, mayonnaise, pickle relish, celery, red onion, mustard, lemon juice, sea salt, garlic powder, Worcestershire sauce, and black pepper. (If desired, cover and chill overnight.) Spoon tuna mixture onto one slice of the bread. Add lettuce. Top with remaining bread slice.

Nutrition Facts per serving: 354 cal., 16 g total fat (3 g sat. fat), 41 mg chol., 964 mg sodium, 29 g carbo., 4 g fibre, 27 g pro.

For WAVE I: Serve the tuna salad in a hollowed pepper instead of using the bread.

*Note: You may substitute 85 g/3 oz of chopped cooked skinless chicken for the tuna.

CHILLI-MINT BURGERS

PREP: 15 MINUTES **GRILL:** 14 MINUTES **MAKES:** 4 SERVINGS

70 g/2½ oz finely chopped onion
1 fresh serrano or jalapeño chilli, seeded and finely chopped,* or
   2 tablespoons bottled diced green chillies
1 tablespoon chopped fresh mint or 1 teaspoon dried mint, crushed
¾ teaspoon ground cumin
1 clove garlic, minced or ⅛ teaspoon garlic powder
¼ teaspoon sea salt
450 g/1 lb lean minced beef or minced turkey breast
2 whole wheat pitta breads, halved
50 g/2 oz Yogurt and Cucumber Sauce (see recipe, page 140)

1. In a medium bowl combine onion, chilli, mint, cumin, garlic, and sea salt. Add the meat; mix well. Shape into four 2-cm/¾-inch-thick patties.

2. Place patties on the rack of a grill or barbecue and grill for 14 to 18 minutes or until meat is done, turning once halfway through grilling.

3. Serve each patty in a pitta half with 1 tablespoon of the Yogurt and Cucumber Sauce.

Nutrition Facts per serving: 361 cal., 19 g total fat (7 g sat. fat), 77 mg chol., 407 mg sodium, 22 g carbo., 3 g fibre, 25 g pro.

*Note: Because chillies contain oils that can burn your skin and eyes, wear rubber or plastic gloves when working with them. If your bare hands do touch the chillies, wash your hands well with soap and water.

GREEN BEAN AND TOMATO SALAD

START TO FINISH: 40 MINUTES **MAKES:** 8 SERVINGS

450 g/1 lb green beans, trimmed
450 g/1 lb cherry tomatoes, halved
1 small red onion, halved crosswise and thinly sliced
1 recipe Red Wine Vinaigrette (see recipe, page 152)
2 tablespoons chopped fresh basil or 2 teaspoons dried basil, crushed
Sea salt
Freshly ground black pepper

1. In a covered medium saucepan cook green beans in a small amount of boiling water for 5 minutes or until crisp-tender. Drain. Submerge in ice water to cool quickly; drain.

2. In a large bowl combine green beans, tomatoes, and onion. Drizzle with Red Wine Vinaigrette; sprinkle with basil. Season to taste with sea salt and black pepper. Toss gently to coat.

Nutrition Facts per serving: 65 cal., 4 g total fat (1 g sat. fat), 0 mg chol., 90 mg sodium, 8 g carbo., 3 g fibre, 2 g pro.

Tip: To serve this as a main-dish salad, add 675 g/1½ lb grilled prawns and/or scallops.

HERB-ROASTED CHICKEN

PREP: 25 MINUTES **CHILL:** 1 TO 24 HOURS **ROAST:** 65 MINUTES
STAND: 10 MINUTES **OVEN:** 230°C/450°F/GAS MARK 8, REDUCING TO
180°C/350°F/GAS MARK 4 **MAKES:** 4 SERVINGS

  12 cloves garlic, minced
  1 tablespoon chopped fresh sage or 1 teaspoon dried sage, crushed
  1 tablespoon chopped fresh rosemary or 1 teaspoon dried rosemary, crushed
  1 tablespoon chopped fresh thyme or 1 teaspoon dried thyme, crushed
  1 1.5 kg/3½ lb whole roasting chicken
  ½ teaspoon sea salt
  ¼ teaspoon freshly ground black pepper
  1 tablespoon extra-virgin olive oil

1. In a small bowl combine garlic and herbs. Sprinkle chicken with sea salt and black pepper. Rub the inside cavity of the chicken with one-third of the herb mixture.

2. Starting at the opening by the leg and thigh, carefully slide your fingertips between the breast meat and the skin to loosen the skin from the meat. Rub the remaining herb mixture between the breast meat and skin and all over the outside of the chicken. With 100% cotton string, tie the ends of the legs together. Twist wing tips under back. Cover and chill the chicken for 1 to 24 hours.

3. Place chicken, breast side down, on a rack set in a shallow roasting pan. Brush oil on the outside of the chicken.

4. Roast in a 230°C/450°F/gas mark 8 oven for 15 minutes; turn chicken breast side up and reduce the oven temperature to 180°C/350°F/gas mark 4. Continue roasting for 50 to 60 minutes more or until drumsticks move easily in their sockets and chicken is no longer pink. Remove chicken from oven. Cover chicken with foil and let stand for 10 minutes before carving. While carving, carefully remove and discard the skin of the chicken.

Nutrition Facts per serving: 261 cal., 9 g total fat (2 g sat. fat), 131 mg chol., 364 mg sodium, 2 g carbo., 0 g fibre, 41 g pro.

CAULIFLOWER WITH PARMESAN CHEESE

PREP: 20 MINUTES **COOK:** 5 MINUTES **MAKES:** 4 SERVINGS

1 675 g/1½ lb cauliflower
2 tablespoons extra-virgin olive oil
⅛ teaspoon crushed red pepper
   Freshly ground black pepper
3 tablespoons chopped fresh flat-leaf parsley
3 tablespoons freshly grated Parmesan cheese
4 lemon wedges

1. Cut cauliflower into florets. In a large frying-pan heat oil over medium heat; add cauliflower and crushed red pepper. Cook and stir for 5 to 8 minutes or until cauliflower is crisp-tender. Remove from heat; season to taste with black pepper. Stir in parsley. Sprinkle with Parmesan. Serve warm or at room temperature (do not let stand at room temperature for more than 2 hours). Pass lemon wedges.

Nutrition Facts per serving: 125 cal., 8 g total fat (2 g sat. fat), 3 mg chol., 112 mg sodium, 12 g carbo., 6 g fibre, 5 g pro.

WILD RICE SALAD WITH CHICKEN

PREP: 20 MINUTES **COOK:** 45 MINUTES **MAKES:** 4 SERVINGS

> 2 tablespoons finely chopped onion or shallots
> 2 tablespoons cider or apple juice
> 1 clove garlic, minced
> 450 ml/¾ pint water
> 140 g/5 oz wild rice, rinsed and drained
> 50 ml/2 fl oz Standard Vinaigrette (see recipe, page 152)
> 2 large Granny Smith apples, cored and chopped
> 1 teaspoon chopped fresh sage or ¼ teaspoon dried sage, crushed
> 340 g/12 oz cooked skinless chicken or turkey breast, sliced
> 25 g/1 oz chopped walnuts, toasted

1. In a large saucepan combine onion, cider, and garlic. Bring to boiling; reduce heat. Cook, uncovered, about 5 minutes or until liquid is evaporated. Add the water. Bring to boiling. Stir in wild rice. Return to boiling; reduce heat. Cover and simmer about 45 minutes or until most of the water is absorbed and wild rice is tender. Drain off excess liquid if necessary.

2. Stir in Standard Vinaigrette until well mixed. Add apples and sage; toss to combine. Serve warm or at room temperature (do not let stand at room temperature for more than 2 hours). Serve sliced chicken on top of salad. Sprinkle with walnuts.

Nutrition Facts per serving: 418 cal., 17 g total fat (3 g sat. fat), 72 mg chol., 140 mg sodium, 34 g carbo., 4 g fibre, 32 g pro.

PORK CHOPS WITH ROSEMARY

PREP: 15 MINUTES **MARINATE:** 1 HOUR **GRILL:** 11 MINUTES
MAKES: 4 SERVINGS

4 pork loin chops (with bone), cut 2 cm/³⁄₄ inch thick
85 ml/3 fl oz dry white wine
1 tablespoon finely shredded lemon peel
85 ml/3 fl oz lemon juice
3 tablespoons extra-virgin olive oil
1 tablespoon chopped fresh rosemary or 1 teaspoon dried rosemary, crushed
¹⁄₂ teaspoon sea salt
¹⁄₄ teaspoon freshly ground black pepper
Fresh rosemary sprigs (optional)

1. Place chops in a self-sealing plastic bag set in a shallow dish. For marinade, in a small bowl combine wine, lemon peel, lemon juice, oil, rosemary, sea salt, and black pepper. Pour over chops. Seal bag; turn to coat chops. Marinate in the refrigerator for 1 hour, turning bag occasionally.

2. Drain chops, discarding marinade. Place chops on the rack of a grill or barbecue and grill for 11 to 13 minutes or until done and juices run clear, turning once halfway through grilling.

Nutrition Facts per serving: 139 cal., 6 g total fat (2 g sat. fat), 47 mg chol., 60 mg sodium, 0 g carbo., 0 g fibre, 19 g pro.

BRUSSELS SPROUTS WITH PROSCIUTTO

START TO FINISH: 20 MINUTES **MAKES:** 4 SERVINGS

340 g/12 oz Brussels sprouts
1 tablespoon extra-virgin olive oil
50 g/2 oz prosciutto or lean cooked ham, chopped
1 teaspoon finely shredded lemon peel
1 tablespoon lemon juice
¼ teaspoon sea salt
⅛ teaspoon freshly ground black pepper

1. Trim stems and remove any wilted outer leaves from Brussels sprouts. Halve any large Brussels sprouts. In a covered large saucepan cook Brussels sprouts in enough boiling lightly salted water to cover for 7 to 9 minutes or just until tender. Drain well.

2. Add oil to same saucepan. Heat over medium-high heat. Add Brussels sprouts, prosciutto, lemon peel, lemon juice, sea salt, and black pepper. Cook and stir for 1 to 2 minutes or until coated and heated through.

Nutrition Facts per serving: 113 cal., 7 g total fat (1 g sat. fat), 0 mg chol., 393 mg sodium, 8 g carbo., 3 g fibre, 6 g pro.

GREEK PIZZA

PREP: 15 MINUTES **BAKE:** 10 MINUTES **OVEN:** 200°C/400°F/GAS MARK 6 **MAKES:** 4 SERVINGS

1 30 cm/12 inch whole wheat pizza base
85 g/3 oz whole fresh baby spinach leaves
225 g/8 oz cooked skinless chicken breast, sliced
70 g/2½ oz cherry tomatoes, quartered
25 g/1 oz crumbled feta cheese
2 tablespoons chopped walnuts or pine nuts
½ teaspoon dried oregano, crushed, or 1½ teaspoons chopped fresh oregano
½ teaspoon dried rosemary, crushed, or 1½ teaspoons chopped fresh rosemary
1 recipe Red Wine Vinaigrette (see recipe, page 152)

1. Place pizza base on a large baking sheet. Top with spinach, chicken, tomatoes, feta cheese, nuts, oregano, and rosemary. Drizzle with Red Wine Vinaigrette. Bake in a 200°C/400°F/gas mark 6 oven for 10 to 15 minutes or until heated through.

Nutrition Facts per serving: 404 cal., 17 g total fat (4 g sat. fat), 56 mg chol., 639 mg sodium, 38 g carbo., 6 g fibre, 29 g pro.

WAVE 1
ADDITIONAL
RECIPES

MARINATED BEEF ROAST

PREP: 20 MINUTES **MARINATE:** 2 TO 3 DAYS **GRILL:** 1½ HOURS
MAKES: 12 TO 14 SERVINGS

>   1 1.5 kg/3 lb boneless beef roast
>   Sea salt (optional)
>   Freshly ground black pepper (optional)
>   565 ml/1 pint water
>   565 ml/1 pint vinegar
>   2 medium onions, sliced
>   1 medium lemon, sliced
>   2 or 3 bay leaves
>   12 whole cloves
>   6 whole black peppercorns
>   1 teaspoon sea salt

1. If desired, season meat with sea salt and black pepper. Place meat in a large self-sealing plastic bag set in a large, deep bowl. For marinade, in a medium bowl combine the water, vinegar, onions, lemon, bay leaves, cloves, peppercorns, and the 1 teaspoon sea salt. Pour over meat. Seal bag; turn to coat meat. Marinate in the refrigerator for 2 to 3 days, turning bag occasionally. Drain meat, reserving marinade.

2. Place meat on the rack of a grill or barbecue and grill for 1½ to 2 hours or until medium doneness, brushing occasionally with reserved marinade during the first hour of grilling. Discard any remaining marinade.

Nutrition Facts per serving: 147 cal., 5 g total fat (2 g sat. fat), 72 mg chol., 83 mg sodium, 0 g carbo., 0 g fibre, 24 g pro.

JERK LONDON GRILL

PREP: 10 MINUTES **MARINATE:** 4 TO 24 HOURS **GRILL:** 17 MINUTES
MAKES: 6 SERVINGS

4 spring onions
50 ml/2 fl oz lime juice
1 2.5-cm/1-inch piece fresh ginger, sliced
½ of a Scotch bonnet chilli, seeded and finely chopped (optional)*
2 tablespoons extra-virgin olive oil
3 cloves garlic
2 teaspoons Jamaican jerk seasoning
1 565 to 675 g/1¼ to 1½ lb beef steak
Sea salt (optional)
Freshly ground black pepper (optional)

1. For marinade, in a blender combine spring onions, lime juice, ginger, chilli (if desired), oil, garlic, and jerk seasoning; cover and blend until smooth. Score both sides of steak in a diamond pattern by making shallow cuts at 2.5-cm/1-inch intervals. If desired, season steak with sea salt and black pepper. Place steak in a glass dish; spread marinade over the steak. Cover dish with clingfilm and marinate in the refrigerator for 4 to 24 hours. Drain steak, discarding marinade.

2. Place steak on the rack of a grill or barbecue and grill for 17 to 21 minutes or until medium doneness, turning once halfway through grilling.

3. To serve, thinly slice meat diagonally across the grain.

Nutrition Facts per serving: 189 cal., 11 g total fat (3 g sat. fat), 47 mg chol., 161 mg sodium, 2 g carbo., 0 g fibre, 20 g pro.

*Note: Because chillies contain oils that can burn your skin and eyes, wear rubber or plastic gloves when working with them. If your bare hands do touch the chillies, wash your hands well with soap and water.

LEMON-GARLIC PORK CHOPS

PREP: 5 MINUTES **MARINATE:** 30 MINUTES **GRILL:** 12 MINUTES
MAKES: 4 SERVINGS

    8 boneless pork loin chops, cut 2 cm/¾ inch thick
    Sea salt (optional)
    Coarsely ground black pepper (optional)
50 ml/2 fl oz extra-virgin olive oil
  1 teaspoon finely shredded lemon peel
50 ml/2 fl oz lemon juice
  1 tablespoon chopped fresh tarragon or 1 teaspoon dried tarragon, crushed
  4 cloves garlic, minced
  ½ teaspoon coarsely ground black pepper

1. If desired, season meat with sea salt and black pepper. Place meat in a self-sealing plastic bag set in a shallow dish. For marinade, combine oil, lemon peel, lemon juice, tarragon, garlic, and the ½ teaspoon pepper. Pour over meat. Seal bag; turn to coat meat. Marinate in the refrigerator for 30 minutes, turning bag occasionally.

2. Drain meat, reserving marinade. Place meat on the rack of a grill or barbecue and grill for 12 to 15 minutes or until done and juices run clear, turning once and brushing with reserved marinade halfway through grilling. Discard any remaining marinade.

Nutrition Facts per serving: 196 cal., 9 g total fat (3 g sat. fat), 62 mg chol., 46 mg sodium, 1 g carbo., 0 g fibre, 25 g pro.

HORSERADISH PORK WRAP

START TO FINISH: 10 MINUTES **MAKES:** 1 SERVING

1 tablespoon Soured Cream-Horseradish Sauce
1 20-cm/8-inch whole wheat flour tortilla
85 g/3 oz leftover Mediterranean Pork Chops* (see recipe, page 173), sliced, or other cooked pork
40 g/1½ oz shredded or torn cos lettuce or whole fresh baby spinach leaves
70 g/2½ oz bite-size red pepper strips

1. Spread Soured Cream-Horseradish Sauce on one side of the tortilla. Top with sliced pork, cos lettuce, and pepper strips. Roll up.

Nutrition Facts per serving: 306 cal., 9 g total fat (3 g sat. fat), 67 mg chol., 598 mg sodium, 23 g carbo., 13 g fibre, 32 g pro.

*Note: If using bone-in pork chops, remove meat from bone.

Soured Cream-Horseradish Sauce: In a small bowl stir together 85 ml/3 fl oz light soured cream and 1 tablespoon prepared horseradish. Makes about eight 1-tablespoon servings.

Nutrition Facts per serving: 14 cal., 1 g total fat (0 g sat. fat), 3 mg chol., 12 mg sodium, 1 g carbo., 0 g fibre, 1 g pro.

TANDOORI CHICKEN SONOMA WRAP

START TO FINISH: 10 MINUTES **MAKES:** 1 SERVING

85 g/3 oz leftover grilled Tandoori Chicken (see recipe, page 177), sliced
40 g/1½ oz shredded or torn cos lettuce or whole fresh baby spinach leaves
50 g/2 oz leftover Roasted Aubergine Salad (see recipe, page 178)
  1 20 cm/8-inch whole wheat flour tortilla
  1 tablespoon Yogurt and Cucumber Sauce (see recipe, page 140)

1. Arrange Tandoori Chicken, cos lettuce, and Roasted Aubergine Salad on the tortilla. Top with Yogurt and Cucumber Sauce. Roll up.

Nutrition Facts per serving: 268 cal., 6 g total fat (1 g sat. fat), 47 mg chol., 488 mg sodium, 23 g carbo., 12 g dietary fibre, 30 g protein.

GARLIC AND MINT CHICKEN BREASTS

PREP: 15 MINUTES **MARINATE:** 4 TO 24 HOURS **GRILL:** 12 MINUTES
MAKES: 4 SERVINGS

6 tablespoons fresh mint leaves
1 tablespoon lemon juice
1 tablespoon extra-virgin olive oil
1 tablespoon soy sauce
1 teaspoon chilli powder
¼ teaspoon freshly ground black pepper
4 cloves garlic
4 skinless, boneless chicken breast halves (565 to 675 g/1¼ to 1½ lb)
Fresh mint sprigs (optional)

1. For marinade, in a blender combine mint leaves, lemon juice, oil, soy sauce, chilli powder, black pepper, and garlic. Cover and blend until smooth.

2. Place chicken in a self-sealing plastic bag set in a shallow dish. Pour marinade over chicken. Seal bag; turn to coat chicken. Marinate in refrigerator for 4 to 24 hours, turning bag occasionally.

3. Drain chicken, discarding marinade. Place chicken on the rack of a grill or barbecue and grill for 12 to 15 minutes or until no longer pink, turning once halfway through grilling.

Nutrition Facts per serving: 202 cal., 6 g total fat (1 g sat. fat), 02 mg chol., 228 mg sodium, 2 g carbo., 0 g fibre, 34 g pro.

PEPPER-LIME CHICKEN

PREP: 10 MINUTES **GRILL:** 25 MINUTES **MAKES:** 6 SERVINGS

900 g to 1.1 kg/2 to 2½ lb chicken breast halves (with bone)
½ teaspoon finely shredded lime peel
50 ml/2 fl oz lime juice
1 tablespoon extra-virgin olive oil
2 cloves garlic, minced
1 tablespoon chopped fresh thyme or basil or 1 teaspoon dried thyme or basil, crushed
½ to 1 teaspoon cracked black pepper
¼ teaspoon sea salt

1. If desired, skin chicken. Place chicken pieces, bone sides up, on the rack of a grill or barbecue and grill for about 20 minutes or until lightly browned.

2. Meanwhile, for glaze, in a bowl stir together lime peel, lime juice, oil, garlic, thyme, black pepper, and sea salt. Brush chicken generously with glaze. Turn chicken; brush generously with glaze. Discard any remaining glaze. Grill for 5 to 15 minutes more or until chicken is no longer pink.

Nutrition Facts per serving: 120 cal., 4 g total fat (1 g sat. fat), 48 mg chol., 126 mg sodium, 1 g carbo., 0 g fibre, 19 g pro.

GRILLED TUNA WITH ROSEMARY

PREP: 10 MINUTES **GRILL:** 8 MINUTES **MAKES:** 4 SERVINGS

450 g/1 lb fresh or frozen tuna, halibut, or salmon steaks, cut 2.5 cm/1 inch thick
2 teaspoons extra-virgin olive oil
2 teaspoons lemon juice
1/8 teaspoon sea salt
1/8 teaspoon freshly ground black pepper
2 cloves garlic, minced
2 teaspoons chopped fresh rosemary or tarragon or 1 teaspoon dried rosemary or tarragon, crushed
1 tablespoon drained capers, slightly crushed
Fresh rosemary sprigs (optional)

1 Thaw fish, if frozen. Rinse fish; pat dry with paper towels. Cut fish into 4 serving-size pieces. Brush both sides of fish with oil and lemon juice; sprinkle with sea salt and black pepper. Sprinkle garlic and rosemary evenly onto fish; rub in with your fingers.

2. Place fish on the greased rack of a grill or barbecue and grill for 8 to 12 minutes or until fish flakes easily when tested with a fork, turning once halfway through grilling.

3. Top fish with capers. If desired, garnish with fresh rosemary.

Nutrition Facts per serving: 145 cal., 3 g total fat (1 g sat. fat), 51 mg chol., 179 mg sodium, 1 g carbo., 0 g fibre, 27 g pro.

ORANGE ROUGHY WITH CORIANDER PESTO

PREP: 20 MINUTES **GRILL:** 4 TO 6 MINUTES PER 1-CM/½-INCH THICKNESS **MAKES:** 4 SERVINGS

450 to 565 g/1 to 1¼ lb fresh or frozen orange roughy or cod fillets
85 g/3 oz loosely packed fresh coriander leaves
1 fresh jalapeño chilli, seeded and chopped*
1 clove garlic, halved
2 tablespoons extra-virgin olive oil
1 tablespoon lime juice
¼ teaspoon sea salt
¼ teaspoon freshly ground black pepper

1. Thaw fish, if frozen. Rinse fish; pat dry with paper towels. Cut fish into 4 serving-size pieces, if necessary. Measure thickness of fish. Set fish aside.

2. For coriander pesto, in a small food processor or blender combine coriander, jalapeño chilli, garlic, 1 tablespoon of the oil, and the lime juice. Cover and process or blend with several on/off turns until almost smooth, stopping the machine and scraping side several times. Set aside.

3. Place fish on the greased rack of a grill, tucking under any thin edges. Brush with remaining 1 tablespoon oil. Sprinkle with sea salt and black pepper. Grill until fish flakes easily when tested with a fork. Allow 4 to 6 minutes per 1-cm/½-inch thickness of fish. If fish is 2.5 cm/1 inch or more thick, turn once halfway through grilling. Serve with coriander pesto.

Nutrition Facts per serving: 148 cal., 8 g total fat (1 g sat. fat), 22 mg chol., 233 mg sodium, 2 g carbo., 1 g fibre, 17 g pro.

*Note: Because chillies contain oils that can burn your skin and eyes, wear rubber or plastic gloves when working with them. If your bare hands do touch the chillies, wash your hands well with soap and water.

PAN-SEARED SCALLOPS WITH LEMON VINAIGRETTE

PREP: 20 MINUTES **COOK:** 6 MINUTES **MAKES:** 4 SERVINGS

340 g/12 oz fresh or frozen sea scallops
1 lemon
450 g/1 lb fresh asparagus spears, cut into 5-cm/2-inch pieces
1 medium red onion, cut into thin wedges
3 tablespoons extra-virgin olive oil
Sea salt (optional)
Freshly ground black pepper (optional)
2 or 3 fresh basil sprigs

1. Thaw scallops, if frozen. Rinse scallops; pat dry with paper towels. Set scallops aside.

2. Score lemon into 4 lengthwise sections with a sharp knife; remove peel from lemon. Scrape off white portion from peel; discard. Cut peel into very thin strips; set aside. Squeeze 2 tablespoons juice from lemon; set juice aside.

3. In a large frying-pan cook asparagus and red onion in 1 tablespoon of the oil for 2 to 3 minutes or until crisp-tender. Season to taste with sea salt and black pepper. Transfer asparagus mixture to a serving platter; keep warm.

4. In the same pan combine reserved lemon peel, the remaining 2 tablespoons oil, and the basil sprigs. Cook for 30 seconds to 1 minute or until heated through. Remove lemon peel and basil sprigs with a slotted spoon, reserving oil in pan. Discard lemon peel and basil sprigs.

5. If desired, season scallops with sea salt and black pepper. Cook scallops in the hot flavoured oil for 3 to 5 minutes or until scallops are opaque, turning once. Stir in reserved lemon juice. Serve scallops with asparagus mixture.

Nutrition Facts per serving: 190 cal., 11 g total fat (1 g sat. fat), 28 mg chol., 147 mg sodium, 6 g carbo., 1 g fibre, 16 g pro.

RED SNAPPER WITH PEPPER AND FENNEL

PREP: 25 MINUTES **BAKE:** 4 MINUTES **OVEN:** 230°C/450°F/
GAS MARK 8 **MAKES:** 4 SERVINGS

450 g/1 lb fresh or frozen skinless red snapper fillets, about 1 cm/½ inch thick
 Sea salt (optional)
 Freshly ground black pepper (optional)
 1 teaspoon fennel seeds, ground
 1 teaspoon finely shredded lemon peel
115 g/4 oz sliced fennel bulb
 70 g/2½ oz chopped onion
 70 g/2½ oz chopped red pepper
 2 cloves garlic, minced
 1 tablespoon extra-virgin olive oil
50 ml/2 fl oz chicken stock
 1 tablespoon chopped fresh dill or 1 teaspoon dried dill
 ¼ teaspoon sea salt
 ¼ teaspoon freshly ground black pepper
 Fresh dill sprigs (optional)

1. Thaw fish, if frozen. Rinse fish; pat dry with paper towels. Cut fish into 4 serving-size pieces, if necessary. If desired, season fish with sea salt and black pepper. Sprinkle fennel seeds and lemon peel evenly onto fish; rub in with your fingers. Set fish aside.

2. In a large frying-pan cook and stir sliced fennel, onion, pepper, and garlic in hot oil over medium heat for 5 to 7 minutes or until vegetables are tender and light brown. Remove from heat. Stir in stock, dill, the ¼ teaspoon sea salt, and the ¼ teaspoon black pepper.

3. Spoon about half the vegetable mixture into a 2.2-litre/4-pint square baking dish. Place fish on top of vegetables; turn under thin edges of fish. Spoon remaining vegetable mixture over top of fish.

4. Bake, uncovered, in a 230°C/450°F/gas mark 8 oven for 4 to 6 minutes or until fish flakes easily when tested with a fork. Transfer fish and vegetables to serving plates. If desired, garnish with dill sprigs.

Nutrition Facts per serving: 157 cal., 5 g total fat (1 g sat. fat), 28 mg chol., 195 mg sodium, 6 g carbo., 2 g fibre, 24 g pro.

THREE-MUSHROOM SOUP

PREP: 15 MINUTES **COOK:** 30 MINUTES **MAKES:** 6 SERVINGS

225 g/8 oz fresh mushrooms, sliced 1 cm/½ inch think
50 g/2 oz fresh portobello mushroom, sliced 1 cm/½ inch thick
50 g/2 oz fresh shiitake, porcini, or other mushrooms, sliced
   1 cm/½ inch thick
70 g/2½ oz chopped onion
  3 cloves garlic, minced
  1 tablespoon extra-virgin olive oil
1.2 litres/2 pints chicken stock
  1 tablespoon chopped fresh thyme or ½ teaspoon dried thyme, crushed

1. In a large saucepan cook mushrooms, onion, and garlic in hot oil about 10 minutes or until mushrooms have softened and most of the liquid has evaporated, stirring occasionally.

2. Add chicken stock and dried thyme (if using). Bring to boiling; reduce heat. Cover and simmer for 20 minutes. Stir in the fresh thyme (if using).

Nutrition Facts per serving: 58 cal., 3 g total fat (0 g sat. fat), 0 mg chol., 474 mg sodium, 5 g carbo., 1 g fibre, 4 g pro.

CHOPPED SALMON SALAD

START TO FINISH: 35 MINUTES **MAKES:** 4 SERVINGS

Non-stick olive oil cooking spray
170 g/6 oz flaked smoked salmon
40 g/1½ oz thinly sliced spring onions
70 g/2½ oz coarsely chopped yellow pepper
200 g/7 oz chopped seeded tomatoes
40 g/1½ oz chopped onion
1 medium cucumber, coarsely chopped
2 tablespoons chopped ripe olives
2 teaspoons small capers, rinsed and drained
1 recipe Lemon Vinaigrette

1. Coat four 170 g/6 oz coffee cups with non-stick cooking spray. Equally divide and layer ingredients in each cup in the following order: salmon, spring onions, pepper, tomatoes, onion, and cucumber. Cover tops with clingfilm and firmly press mixture into cups with a soup can or similar object slightly smaller than diameter of cup.

2. To serve, invert salads onto 4 salad plates; carefully lift off cups. Sprinkle salads with olives and capers; drizzle with Lemon Vinaigrette.

Lemon Vinaigrette: In a screw-top jar combine 2 tablespoons extra-virgin olive oil, 2 teaspoons finely shredded lemon peel, 2 tablespoons lemon juice, sugar substitute to equal ½ teaspoon sugar, ¼ teaspoon sea salt, and several dashes bottled hot pepper sauce. Shake well before serving.

Nutrition Facts per serving: 135 cal., 9 g total fat (1 g sat. fat), 7 mg chol., 429 mg sodium, 9 g carbo., 2 g fibre, 7 g pro.

Soy-Sauced Broccoli and Peppers

START TO FINISH: 20 MINUTES **MAKES:** 4 SERVINGS

3 tablespoons soy sauce
1 tablespoon lemon juice
1 teaspoon grated fresh ginger
1 clove garlic, minced
1 teaspoon toasted sesame oil
450 g/1 lb broccoli florets
2 medium red and/or yellow peppers, cut into strips
1 tablespoon chopped fresh coriander

1. For sauce, stir together soy sauce, lemon juice, ginger, garlic, and sesame oil; set aside.

2. Place steamer basket in a very large pan. Add water to just below the bottom of the steamer basket. Bring water to boiling. Place broccoli in steamer basket. Reduce heat; cover and steam for 4 minutes. Add the peppers; cover and steam for 3 to 4 minutes more or until vegetables are crisp-tender. Drain vegetables; transfer vegetables to a serving bowl. Drizzle sauce over vegetables, tossing gently to coat. Sprinkle with coriander.

Nutrition Facts per serving: 30 cal., 1 g total fat (0 g sat. fat), 0 mg chol., 246 mg sodium, 5 g carbo., 2 g fibre, 0 g pro.

WAVES 2 AND 3 ADDITIONAL RECIPES

SUMMER SQUASH COMBO

START TO FINISH: 20 MINUTES **MAKES:** 6 SERVINGS

- 2 tablespoons white or red wine vinegar
- 2 tablespoons extra-virgin olive oil
- 2 teaspoons chopped fresh oregano or thyme or ½ teaspoon dried oregano or thyme, crushed
- 1 teaspoon finely shredded lemon peel
- ¼ teaspoon sea salt
- ⅛ to ¼ teaspoon crushed red pepper
- 3 spring onions, trimmed
- 1 medium courgette, quartered lengthwise
- 1 medium yellow pattypan squash, quartered lengthwise

1. In a small bowl stir together vinegar, oil, oregano, lemon peel, sea salt, and crushed red pepper. Brush spring onions, courgette, and yellow pattypan squash with some of the vinegar mixture.

2. Place vegetables on the rack of a grill or barbecue and grill until crisp-tender, turning occasionally. Allow 3 to 4 minutes for spring onions and 5 to 6 minutes for courgette and yellow pattypan squash.

3. Cut grilled vegetables into bite-size pieces; transfer to a serving bowl. Toss with remaining vinegar mixture. Serve warm.

Nutrition Facts per serving: 51 cal., 5 g total fat (1 g sat. fat), 0 mg chol., 101 mg sodium, 2 g carbo., 1 g fibre, 1 g pro.

CHEESY VEGETABLE EGGS

PREP: 20 MINUTES **BAKE:** 20 MINUTES **STAND:** 5 MINUTES
OVEN: 180°C/350°F/GAS MARK 4 **MAKES:** 4 SERVINGS

>   1 tablespoon extra-virgin olive oil
>   1 teaspoon chopped fresh thyme
>   1 clove garlic, minced
> 275 g/10 oz chopped onion, chopped pepper, sliced button mushrooms,
>   seeded and chopped tomatoes, and/or chopped courgettes
>   ¼ teaspoon sea salt
>   ⅛ teaspoon freshly ground black pepper
>   Non-stick olive oil cooking spray
>   8 eggs
>   1 tablespoon chopped fresh chives or parsley
>   85 g/3 oz grated reduced-fat Swiss, mozzarella, or Cheddar cheese

1. In a medium non-stick frying-pan heat the olive oil over medium heat. Add thyme and garlic; cook for 10 seconds. Stir in vegetables; cook and stir for 3 to 4 minutes or until vegetables are tender. Sprinkle with sea salt and black pepper; set vegetables aside.

2. Coat a 3.4-litre/6-pint rectangular baking dish with non-stick cooking spray. Spread cooked vegetable mixture evenly over the bottom of the prepared dish. Carefully break eggs into pan on top of vegetables. Sprinkle with chives and, if desired, additional sea salt and black pepper.

3. Bake, covered, in a 180°C/350°F/gas mark 4 oven about 20 minutes or until egg whites are opaque and yolks are firm. Sprinkle cheese over eggs. Cover and let stand about 5 minutes or until cheese is melted.

Nutrition Facts per serving: 230 cal., 15 g total fat (4 g sat. fat), 429 mg chol., 311 mg sodium, 6 g carbo., 1 g fibre, 19 g pro.

Scrambled Eggs with Feta and Dill

START TO FINISH: 25 MINUTES **MAKES:** 4 SERVINGS

    1 tablespoon extra-virgin olive oil
    8 slices prosciutto or lean ham
    8 eggs
   50 ml/2 fl oz water
115 g/4 oz crumbled feta cheese
    1 tablespoon chopped fresh dill or 1 teaspoon dried dill
    ⅛ teaspoon freshly ground black pepper
      Non-stick olive oil cooking spray

1. Heat the oil in a large non-stick frying-pan over medium heat. Add prosciutto or ham and cook for 4 to 6 minutes or until light brown, turning once. Transfer to plate; cover and keep warm. Rinse and dry pan.

2. In a medium bowl whisk together eggs, water, feta cheese, dill, and black pepper.

3. Coat the frying-pan with non-stick cooking spray. Heat over medium heat; pour in egg mixture. Cook, without stirring, until mixture begins to set on the bottom and around edge. With a spatula or a large spoon, lift and fold the partially cooked egg mixture so that the uncooked portion flows underneath. Continue cooking until egg mixture is cooked through but is still glossy and moist. Remove from heat. Serve with prosciutto or ham.

Nutrition Facts per serving: 344 cal., 24 g total fat (10 g sat. fat), 483 mg chol., 1,192 mg sodium, 3 g carbo., 0 g fibre, 28 g pro.

SMOKED SALMON FRITTATA

START TO FINISH: 25 MINUTES **MAKES:** 4 SERVINGS

6 eggs
¼ teaspoon freshly ground black pepper
   Non-stick olive oil cooking spray
40 g/1½ oz sliced spring onions
   1 115 g/4 oz piece smoked salmon, flaked, with skin and bones removed
   2 tablespoons chopped fresh dill or 1 teaspoon dried dill
   1 25 g/1 oz semi-soft goat's cheese, crumbled

1. In a medium bowl combine eggs and black pepper; set aside.

2. Lightly coat a large frying-pan with cooking spray. Cook onions in pan over medium heat until tender. Stir in salmon and dill. Pour egg mixture into pan over salmon. As mixture sets, run a spatula around edge of pan, lifting egg mixture so the uncooked portion flows underneath. Continue cooking and lifting edges until almost set (surface will be moist).

3. Place pan under the grill 10 to 12 cm/4 to 5 inches from the heat. Grill for 1 to 2 minutes or until top is just set. Sprinkle with goat's cheese.

Nutrition Facts per serving: 166 cal., 10 g total fat (4 g sat. fat), 329 mg chol., 344 mg sodium, 1 g carbo., 0 g fibre, 16 g pro.

GARLIC-MUSTARD STEAK

PREP: 10 MINUTES **GRILL:** 15 MINUTES **MAKES:** 4 TO 6 SERVINGS

1 450 to 675 g/1 to 1½ lb beef steak
Sea salt (optional)
Coarsely ground black pepper (optional)
2 tablespoons Dijon-style mustard
1 tablespoon Worcestershire sauce
1 tablespoon chopped fresh marjoram or thyme or ½ teaspoon dried marjoram
or thyme, crushed
2 cloves garlic, minced
¼ teaspoon coarsely ground black pepper

1. Score both sides of steak in a diamond pattern by making shallow diagonal cuts at 2.5-cm/ 1-inch intervals. If desired, season steak with sea salt and black pepper. In a small bowl combine mustard, Worcestershire sauce, marjoram, garlic, and the ¼ teaspoon black pepper. Brush both sides of steak with mustard mixture.

2. Grill the meat for 15 to 18 minutes or until medium doneness, turning once halfway through grilling. Thinly slice meat diagonally across the grain.

Nutrition Facts per serving: 183 cal., 8 g total fat (3 g sat. fat), 56 mg chol., 360 mg sodium, 3 g carbo., 0 g fibre, 25 g pro.

BURGERS WITH DILL SAUCE

PREP: 20 MINUTES **GRILL:** 12 MINUTES **MAKES:** 4 SERVINGS

    40 g/1½ oz finely chopped onion
     3 tablespoons chopped fresh parsley
    ½ teaspoon sea salt
     6 cloves garlic, minced
    450 g/1 lb lean minced beef or lamb
     50 ml/2 fl oz low-fat soured cream or plain low-fat yogurt
     2 tablespoons mayonnaise
     1 tablespoon Dijon-style mustard or whole grain brown mustard
     1 teaspoon chopped fresh dill or ¼ teaspoon dried dill
     1 teaspoon balsamic vinegar
    40 g/1½ oz chopped, seeded cucumber

1. In a large bowl combine onion, parsley, sea salt, and garlic. Add meat; mix well. Shape into four 2-cm/¾-inch-thick patties.

2. Grill the patties for 12 to 14 minutes or until done, turning once halfway through grilling.

3. Meanwhile, for sauce, in a small bowl combine soured cream, mayonnaise, mustard, dill, and vinegar. Stir in cucumber. Spoon sauce over burgers.

Nutrition Facts per serving: 304 cal., 22 g total fat (8 g sat. fat), 82 mg chol., 491 mg sodium, 3 g carbo., 0 g fibre, 23 g pro.

PORK CHOPS WITH CURRY MARINADE

PREP: 15 MINUTES **MARINATE:** 6 TO 24 HOURS **GRILL:** 20 MINUTES
MAKES: 4 SERVINGS

115 g/4 oz spicy brown mustard
50 ml/2 fl oz dry white wine
1 tablespoon curry powder
1 tablespoon extra-virgin olive oil
2 tablespoons sliced spring onion
1 teaspoon grated fresh ginger
1 clove garlic, minced
¼ to ½ teaspoon crushed red pepper
4 boneless pork loin chops, cut 2.5 cm/1 inch thick (about 450 g/1 lb total)
   Sea salt (optional)
   Freshly ground black pepper (optional)

1. For marinade, in a small bowl stir together mustard, wine, curry powder, oil, spring onion, ginger, garlic, and crushed red pepper.

2. If desired, season chops with sea salt and black pepper. Place chops in a self-sealing plastic bag set in a shallow dish. Pour marinade over chops. Seal bag; turn to coat chops. Marinate in the refrigerator for 6 to 24 hours, turning bag occasionally.

3. Drain chops, reserving marinade. Place chops on the rack of a grill or barbecue and grill for 20 to 24 minutes or until done and juices run clear, turning once and brushing with marinade halfway through grilling. Discard any remaining marinade.

Nutrition Facts per serving: 191 cal., 12 g total fat (3 g sat. fat), 51 mg chol., 343 mg sodium, 2 g carbo., 1 g fibre, 18 g pro.

GREEK-STUFFED ROASTED PORK LOIN

PREP: 25 MINUTES **ROAST:** 1 HOUR **STAND:** 15 MINUTES
OVEN: 170°C/325°F/GAS MARK 3 **MAKES:** 8 SERVINGS

> 1 900 g to 1.1 kg/2 to 2½ lb boneless pork top loin roast (single loin)
> Sea salt
> Freshly ground black pepper
> 1½ teaspoons dried oregano
> 1 340 g/12 oz jar roasted red peppers, drained
> 50 g/2 oz crumbled feta cheese
> 2 cloves garlic, minced
> Steamed kale (optional)

1. To butterfly the pork roast, make a lengthwise cut down the centre of the roast, cutting to within 1 cm/½ inch of the opposite side, forming a "v." Spread open. Make a parallel slit on each side of the original cut. Open meat to lie flat. Place between 2 pieces of clingfilm. Working from centre to edges, pound with the flat side of a meat mallet to 1-cm/½-inch thickness. Remove clingfilm. Season meat with sea salt and black pepper.

2. Sprinkle oregano on pounded side of pork loin. Remove and discard any seeds in roasted peppers. If necessary, split peppers to lie flat. Arrange peppers in an even layer on top of the meat. In a small bowl combine feta cheese and garlic. Sprinkle over peppers on pork loin. Starting from a short side, roll up pork; tie with 100% cotton string at 3.5-cm/ 1½-inch intervals. Sprinkle with additional sea salt and black pepper.

3. Place roast on a rack in a shallow roasting pan. Roast in a 170°C/325°F/gas mark 3 oven for 1 to 1½ hours. Cover roast with foil and let stand for 15 minutes. If desired, serve with steamed kale.

Nutrition Facts per serving: 196 cal., 8 g total fat (3 g sat. fat), 68 mg chol., 171 mg sodium, 2 g carbo., 1 g fibre, 26 g pro.

SPICE-ROASTED CHICKEN

PREP: 25 MINUTES **ROAST:** 1¼ HOURS **STAND:** 10 MINUTES
OVEN: 230°C/450°F/GAS MARK 8, REDUCING TO 180°C/350°F/GAS
MARK 4 **MAKES:** 4 SERVINGS

12 cloves garlic, minced
4 teaspoons fennel seeds, toasted and ground,*
   or 4 teaspoons ground fennel seeds
4 teaspoons paprika
2 teaspoons cumin seeds, toasted and ground,*
   or 2 teaspoons ground cumin
1 tablespoon extra-virgin olive oil
1 1.5 kg/3½ lb whole roasting chicken
½ teaspoon sea salt
⅛ teaspoon freshly ground black pepper
1 small lemon or orange, quartered

1. In a small bowl combine garlic, ground fennel, paprika, and ground cumin. Stir in oil. Sprinkle chicken with sea salt and black pepper. Rub the inside cavity of the chicken with one-third of the garlic mixture.

2. Starting at the opening by the leg and thigh, carefully slide your fingertips between the breast meat and the skin to loosen the skin from the meat. Rub the remaining garlic mixture between the breast meat and skin and all over the outside of the chicken. Place the lemon or orange quarters in the cavity of the chicken. With 100% cotton string, tie the ends of the legs together. Twist wing tips under back. If desired, cover and chill the chicken for up to 24 hours.

3. Transfer the chicken, breast side down, to a rack set in a shallow roasting pan.

4. Roast in a 230°C/450°F/gas mark 8 oven for 15 minutes; turn chicken breast side up and reduce the oven temperature to 180°C/350°F/gas mark 4. Continue roasting for 60 to 70 minutes more or until drumsticks move easily in their sockets and chicken is no longer pink. Remove chicken from oven. Cover chicken with foil and let stand for 10 minutes before carving. While carving, carefully remove and discard the skin of the chicken.

Nutrition Facts per serving: 276 cal., 9 g total fat (2 g sat. fat), 131 mg chol., 368 mg sodium, 4 g carbo., 2 g fibre, 42 g pro.

*Note: To toast seeds, heat a small frying-pan over medium heat. Add seeds. Cook about 2 minutes or until toasted and aromatic, shaking pan frequently. Place toasted seeds in a spice grinder and process until finely ground.

GRILLED CHICKEN WITH TOMATO-BEAN SALAD

PREP: 25 MINUTES **MARINATE:** 8 TO 24 HOURS **GRILL:** 12 MINUTES
MAKES: 4 SERVINGS

    4 115 g/4 oz skinless, boneless chicken breast halves
      Sea salt
      Freshly ground black pepper
   85 g/3 oz Chermoula Marinade (see recipe, page 138)
    2 medium green and/or red peppers, seeded and chopped
    1 400 g/14 oz can chickpeas, rinsed and drained
    1 large tomato, chopped
   70 g/2½ oz finely chopped onion
   ½ of a fresh serrano chilli, seeded and finely chopped* (optional)
    2 tablespoons chopped fresh flat-leaf parsley

1. Season chicken with sea salt and black pepper. Place chicken in a self-sealing plastic bag set in a shallow dish; add a third of the Chermoula Marinade. Seal bag; turn to coat chicken. Marinate in the refrigerator for 8 to 24 hours, turning bag occasionally.

2. Drain chicken, discarding marinade. Place chicken on the rack of a grill or barbecue and grill for 12 to 15 minutes or until chicken is no longer pink, turning once halfway through grilling.

3. Meanwhile, in large bowl combine peppers, chickpeas, tomato, onion, serrano chilli (if desired), and remaining Chermoula Marinade. Season to taste with sea salt and black pepper. Divide chickpea mixture among 4 serving plates. Add a chicken breast half to each plate. Sprinkle with parsley.

Nutrition Facts per serving: 433 cal., 19 g total fat (3 g sat. fat), 66 mg chol., 907 mg sodium, 34 g carbo., 8 g fibre, 33 g pro.

*Note: Because chillies contain oils that can burn your skin and eyes, wear rubber or plastic gloves when working with them. If your bare hands do touch the chillies, wash your hands well with soap and water.

BISTRO CHICKEN AND GARLIC

PREP: 20 MINUTES **BAKE:** 12 MINUTES **OVEN:** 200°C/400°F/GAS MARK 6 **MAKES:** 4 SERVINGS

1 head garlic
4 skinless, boneless chicken breast halves (565 to 675 g/1¼ to 1½ lb total)
   Sea salt (optional)
   Freshly ground black pepper (optional)
1 tablespoon extra-virgin olive oil
1 teaspoon chopped fresh basil or ¼ teaspoon dried basil, crushed
1 teaspoon chopped fresh thyme or ¼ teaspoon dried thyme, crushed
1 teaspoon chopped fresh rosemary or ¼ teaspoon dried rosemary, crushed
¼ teaspoon sea salt
⅛ teaspoon freshly ground black pepper
50 ml/2 fl oz dry vermouth or dry white wine
   Fresh herb sprigs (optional)

1. Separate cloves of garlic, discarding small papery cloves in centre. Trim off stem end of each garlic clove but do not peel. Set aside.

2. If desired, season chicken with sea salt and black pepper. In a large ovenproof frying-pan cook chicken and garlic cloves in hot oil over medium-high heat about 4 minutes or until chicken is light brown, turning chicken and stirring garlic cloves once. Sprinkle chicken with basil, thyme, rosemary, the ¼ teaspoon sea salt, and the ⅛ teaspoon black pepper.

3. Transfer frying-pan to 200°C/400°F/gas mark 6 oven. Bake, covered, for 12 to 15 minutes or until chicken is no longer pink and garlic is tender.

4. Using a slotted spatula, transfer chicken to a serving platter; keep warm. Reserve juices in pan. Transfer garlic cloves to a small bowl; set aside for 1 to 2 minutes to cool slightly. Add vermouth to juices in pan. Squeeze softened garlic from skins into pan; discard skins. Bring to boiling; reduce heat. Simmer, uncovered, about 6 minutes or until sauce thickens slightly, stirring frequently. Pour garlic sauce over chicken. Season to taste with additional sea salt and black pepper. If desired, garnish with herb sprigs.

Nutrition Facts per serving: 177 cal., 7 g total fat (1 g sat. fat), 60 mg chol., 189 mg sodium, 3 g carbo., 0 g fibre, 22 g pro.

CHICKEN AND ASPARAGUS SAUTÉ

START TO FINISH: 20 MINUTES **MAKES:** 4 SERVINGS

340 g/12 oz fresh asparagus spears
4 skinless, boneless chicken breast halves (565 to 675 g/1¼ to 1½ lb total)
2 to 3 teaspoons herbes de Provence or Cajun seasoning
3 cloves garlic, minced
¼ teaspoon sea salt
¼ teaspoon freshly ground black pepper
2 teaspoons extra-virgin olive oil
1 medium red pepper, seeded and cut into thin strips
115 ml/4 fl oz dry white wine or chicken stock
1 tablespoon chopped fresh flat-leaf parsley
1 tablespoon lemon juice

1. Snap off and discard woody base from asparagus. Bias-slice asparagus into 2.5-cm/1-inch pieces; set aside.

2. Sprinkle chicken with herbes de Provence, garlic, sea salt, and black pepper. In a large non-stick frying-pan cook chicken in hot oil over medium-high heat for 3 minutes.

3. Turn chicken; add asparagus, pepper strips, and wine. Bring to boiling; reduce heat. Simmer, uncovered, about 8 minutes or until chicken is no longer pink and vegetables are crisp-tender, stirring vegetables occasionally. Using a slotted spoon, transfer chicken and vegetables to serving plates. Stir parsley and lemon juice into cooking juices in pan. Season to taste with additional sea salt and black pepper. Spoon over chicken.

Nutrition Facts per serving: 223 cal., 5 g total fat (1 g sat. fat), 82 mg chol., 202 mg sodium, 5 g carbo., 2 g fibre, 35 g pro.

CORIANDER CHICKEN WITH NUTS

START TO FINISH: 25 MINUTES **MAKES:** 4 SERVINGS

2 teaspoons grated fresh ginger

4 cloves garlic, minced

¼ teaspoon sea salt

⅛ teaspoon freshly ground black pepper

450 g/1 lb skinless, boneless chicken breasts, cut into 2.5-cm/1-inch strips

2 teaspoons roasted peanut oil

25 g/1 oz dry roasted peanuts

1 tablespoon soy sauce

2 teaspoons rice vinegar

1 teaspoon toasted sesame oil

50 g/2 oz fresh coriander leaves

170 g/6 oz finely shredded Chinese leaves

3 tablespoons chopped fresh mint

Fresh coriander sprigs (optional)

Lime wedges (optional)

1. In a small bowl combine ginger, garlic, sea salt, and black pepper. Sprinkle garlic mixture over chicken; toss to coat. In a heavy 25-cm/10-inch frying-pan cook and stir chicken in hot peanut oil over high heat for 2 minutes. Add peanuts. Cook and stir about 3 minutes more or until chicken is no longer pink.

2. Add soy sauce, vinegar, and sesame oil. Cook and stir for 2 minutes more. Remove from heat. Stir in half the coriander leaves.

3. In a large bowl toss together cabbage, mint, and remaining coriander leaves. Arrange cabbage mixture on a serving platter or 4 serving plates. To serve, spoon chicken mixture over cabbage mixture. If desired, garnish with coriander sprigs and lime wedges.

Nutrition Facts per serving: 217 cal., 8 g total fat (1 g sat. fat), 66 mg chol., 402 mg sodium, 7 g carbo., 2 g fibre, 30 g pro.

STUFFED TURKEY BREASTS

PREP: 15 MINUTES **GRILL:** 16 MINUTES **MAKES:** 4 SERVINGS

2 turkey breasts (about 450 g/1 lb total)
85 g/3 oz chopped fresh spinach
85 g/3 oz semi-soft goat's cheese or crumbled feta cheese
½ teaspoon freshly ground black pepper
1 tablespoon extra-virgin olive oil
1 teaspoon paprika
½ teaspoon sea salt
⅛ to ¼ teaspoon cayenne pepper

1. Make a pocket in each turkey tenderloin by cutting lengthwise from one side almost to, but not through, the opposite side; set aside. In a medium bowl combine spinach, cheese, and black pepper. Divide spinach mixture between pockets. Tie 100% cotton string around each turkey breast in 3 or 4 places to hold in stuffing.

2. In a small bowl combine oil, paprika, sea salt, and cayenne pepper; brush evenly over turkey breasts. Place the turkey on the greased rack of a grill or barbecue and grill for 16 to 20 minutes or until no longer pink, turning once halfway through grilling. Remove and discard strings; slice turkey crosswise.

Nutrition Facts per serving: 219 cal., 9 g total fat (4 g sat. fat), 80 mg chol., 373 mg sodium, 1 g carbo., 1 g fibre, 32 g pro.

SPICED TURKEY BREASTS

PREP: 15 MINUTES **GRILL:** 12 MINUTES **MAKES:** 4 SERVINGS

> **2 turkey breasts (about 450 g/1 lb total)**
> **1½ teaspoons ground cumin**
> **1½ teaspoons coriander seeds, crushed**
> **1 teaspoon finely shredded lime peel**
> **¾ teaspoon sea salt**
> **¾ teaspoon ground ginger**
> **½ teaspoon crushed red pepper**
> **115 ml/4 fl oz plain low-fat yogurt**
> **2 tablespoons lime juice**

1. Cut turkey breasts in half horizontally to make 4 steaks; set aside. In a small bowl combine cumin, coriander seeds, lime peel, sea salt, ginger, and crushed red pepper. Set aside ½ teaspoon of the cumin mixture. Sprinkle remaining cumin mixture evenly over turkey steaks; rub in with your fingers.

2. Place the turkey on the rack of a grill or barbecue and grill for 12 to 15 minutes or until no longer pink, turning once halfway through grilling.

3. Meanwhile, in a small bowl combine yogurt, lime juice, and the reserved cumin mixture. Serve sauce with grilled turkey steaks.

Nutrition Facts per serving: 158 cal., 2 g total fat (1 g sat. fat), 70 mg chol., 439 mg sodium, 4 g carbo., 1 g fibre, 29 g pro.

GRILLED BASS WITH STRAWBERRY SALSA

START TO FINISH: 30 MINUTES **MAKES:** 4 SERVINGS

4 115 to 150 g/4 to 5 oz fresh or frozen sea bass or halibut steaks, 2.5 cm/
    1 inch thick
1 small lime
¼ teaspoon sea salt
¼ teaspoon cayenne pepper
115 g/4 oz chopped strawberries
40 g/1½ oz finely chopped seeded fresh poblano chilli*
2 tablespoons chopped fresh coriander
½ teaspoon cumin seeds, toasted
⅛ teaspoon sea salt

1. Thaw fish, if frozen. Rinse fish; pat dry with paper towels. Finely grate lime peel. Peel, section, and chop lime; set aside. In a small bowl combine lime peel, the ¼ teaspoon sea salt, and the cayenne pepper. Sprinkle evenly onto both sides of fish; rub in with your fingers.

2. Place fish on the greased rack of a grill or barbecue and grill for 14 to 18 minutes or until fish flakes easily when tested with a fork, gently turning once halfway through grilling.

3. Meanwhile, in a medium bowl combine chopped lime, strawberries, poblano chilli, coriander, cumin seeds, and the ⅛ teaspoon sea salt. Serve with grilled fish.

Nutrition Facts per serving: 137 cal., 3 g total fat (1 g sat. fat), 46 mg chol., 299 mg sodium, 7 g carbo., 1 g fibre, 22 g pro.

*Note: Because chillies contain oils that can burn your skin and eyes, wear rubber or plastic gloves when working with them. If your bare hands do touch the chillies, wash your hands well with soap and water.

SEARED TUNA WITH CITRUS RELISH

PREP: 20 MINUTES **COOK:** 6 MINUTES **MAKES:** 4 SERVINGS

    4 115 g/4 oz fresh or frozen tuna steaks, 2 cm/¾ inch thick
    Sea salt (optional)
    Freshly ground black pepper (optional)
    2 teaspoons sherry vinegar or white wine vinegar
    2 teaspoons soy sauce
    ½ teaspoon grated fresh ginger
    1 tablespoon extra-virgin olive oil
    1 medium grapefruit, peeled and sectioned
    1 medium orange, peeled and sliced
    2 tablespoons finely chopped red onion
    2 tablespoons chopped fresh coriander
    2 teaspoons extra-virgin olive oil

1. Thaw fish, if frozen. Rinse fish; pat dry with paper towels. If desired, season fish with sea salt and black pepper. Set aside.

2. For citrus relish, in a small bowl combine vinegar, soy sauce, and ginger. Whisk in the 1 tablespoon oil. Cut grapefruit sections into thirds and coarsely chop orange slices. Stir fruit pieces, red onion, and coriander into vinegar mixture. Set aside.

3. In a large frying-pan heat the 2 teaspoons oil over medium-high heat. Add fish and cook for 6 to 9 minutes or just until fish flakes easily when tested with a fork (tuna can be slightly pink in centre), turning once. Serve the fish with citrus relish.

Nutrition Facts per serving: 244 cal., 11 g total fat (2 g sat. fat), 43 mg chol., 199 mg sodium, 7 g carbo., 1 g fibre, 27 g pro.

POACHED SALMON WITH DILLED SOURED CREAM

PREP: 10 MINUTES **COOK:** 4 MINUTES **CHILL:** 2 TO 24 HOURS
MAKES: 6 SERVINGS

675 g/1½ lb fresh or frozen skinless salmon fillets, about 1 cm/½ inch thick
⅛ teaspoon sea salt
⅛ teaspoon ground white pepper
170 ml/6 fl oz dry white wine
85 ml/3 fl oz water
½ of a lemon, cut into thick slices
1 teaspoon coriander seeds
3 star anise or ½ teaspoon anise seeds
115 ml/4 fl oz low-fat soured cream
1 tablespoon chopped fresh dill
1 tablespoon lime juice
Sea salt
Freshly ground black pepper
1 head Iceberg lettuce, torn into large pieces
Cucumber slices (optional)
Fresh dill sprigs (optional)

1. Thaw fish, if frozen. Rinse fish; pat dry with paper towels. Cut into 6 serving-size pieces, if necessary. Sprinkle fish with the ⅛ teaspoon salt salt and the white pepper.

2. In a large frying-pan combine wine, the water, lemon slices, coriander seeds, and star anise. Bring to boiling; reduce heat. Add fish in a single layer. Cover and simmer for 4 to 6 minutes or until fish flakes easily when tested with a fork. Using a slotted spatula, carefully transfer fish to a platter. Cover and chill for 2 to 24 hours.

3. In a small bowl combine soured cream, chopped dill, and lime juice. Add sea salt and black pepper to taste. Cover and chill for 1 hour or until serving time.

4. Arrange lettuce on 6 serving plates. Top with fish. Spoon soured cream mixture over fish. If desired, garnish with cucumber slices and dill sprigs.

Nutrition Facts per serving: 259 cal., 14 g total fat (3 g sat. fat), 73 mg chol., 143 mg sodium, 4 g carbo., 1 g fibre, 24 g pro.

HALIBUT WITH PEPPER SALSA

PREP: 25 MINUTES **GRILL:** 4 TO 6 MINUTES PER 1-CM/½-INCH
THICKNESS **MAKES:** 4 SERVINGS

    3 tablespoons rice vinegar
    2 tablespoons soy sauce
    ½ teaspoon grated fresh ginger
    ⅛ teaspoon freshly ground black pepper
    115 g/4 oz coarsely chopped red and/or yellow pepper
    50 g/2 oz chopped, seeded cucumber
    2 tablespoons thinly sliced spring onion
    2 tablespoons chopped fresh coriander
    ½ of a small fresh jalapeño chilli, seeded and finely chopped*
    1 teaspoon toasted sesame oil
    4 115 g/4 oz fresh or frozen halibut steaks, 2 to 2.5-cm/¾ to 1 inch thick
    1 teaspoon sesame seeds
    Chinese leaves (optional)

1. For pepper salsa, in a small bowl combine vinegar, soy sauce, and ginger. In another small bowl combine 2 tablespoons of the vinegar mixture and the black pepper; set aside. To the remaining vinegar mixture, add pepper, cucumber, spring onion, coriander, chilli, and sesame oil; toss to coat. Cover and chill until serving time or up to 1 hour.

2. Thaw fish, if frozen. Rinse fish; pat dry with paper towels. Place fish on the greased rack of a grill. Brush steaks with the reserved 2 tablespoons vinegar mixture. Sprinkle with sesame seeds. Grill for 4 to 6 minutes per 1-cm/½-inch thickness or until fish flakes easily when tested with a fork. (If steaks are 2.5 cm/1 inch thick, turn once halfway through grilling.) If desired, line serving plates with cabbage leaves. Place fish on cabbage leaves and serve with pepper salsa.

Nutrition Facts per serving: 150 cal., 3 g total fat (0 g sat. fat), 36 mg chol., 525 mg sodium, 3 g carbo., 1 g fibre, 25 g pro.

*Note: Because chillies contain oils that can burn your skin and eyes, wear rubber or plastic gloves when working with them. If your bare hands do touch the chillies, wash your hands well with soap and water.

PRAWNS WITH COURGETTES AND ASPARAGUS

START TO FINISH: 30 MINUTES **MAKES:** 4 SERVINGS

225 g/8 oz fresh or frozen peeled and deveined medium prawns
   Sea salt (optional)
   Freshly ground black pepper (optional)
5 small courgettes
225 g/8 oz fresh asparagus spears
   1 fresh jalapeño chilli, seeded and finely chopped*
   1 tablespoon grated fresh ginger
   2 cloves garlic, minced
   2 tablespoons extra-virgin olive oil
   2 tablespoons chopped fresh coriander
   1 tablespoon sesame seeds, toasted
   2 teaspoons toasted sesame oil
¼ teaspoon sea salt
¼ teaspoon freshly ground black pepper
   Chopped fresh coriander (optional)
   Sesame seeds, toasted (optional)

1. Thaw prawns, if frozen. Rinse prawns; pat dry with paper towels. If desired, season prawns with sea salt and black pepper. Set aside.

2. Halve each courgette lengthwise. Place each courgette half, cut side down, on a board and cut into long, thin strips. Set aside. Snap off and discard woody bases from asparagus. Cut asparagus diagonally into 2.5-cm/1-inch pieces.

3. Place steamer basket in a large pan. Add water to just below the bottom of the steamer basket. Bring water to boiling. Place asparagus in steamer basket. Cover and steam for 2 minutes; add courgettes and steam for 2 to 3 minutes more or until vegetables are just crisp-tender (don't overcook). Drain well; keep warm.

4. Meanwhile, in a large frying-pan cook jalapeño chilli, ginger, and garlic in hot oil over medium-high heat for 30 seconds. Add prawns. Cook for 2 to 3 minutes or until prawns are opaque, stirring often. Stir in the 2 tablespoons chopped coriander, sesame seeds, sesame oil, the ¼ teaspoon sea salt, and the ¼ teaspoon black pepper. Add courgettes and asparagus to pan; toss gently to coat. Transfer to a serving platter. If desired, sprinkle with additional chopped coriander and/or sesame seeds.

Nutrition Facts per serving: 186 cal., 11 g total fat (2 g sat. fat), 86 mg chol., 221 mg sodium, 8 g carbo., 3 g fibre, 14 g pro.

*Note: Because chillies contain oils that can burn your skin and eyes, wear rubber or plastic gloves when working with them. If your bare hands do touch the chillies, wash your hands well with soap and water.

HAM AND LENTIL SOUP

PREP: 35 MINUTES **COOK:** 1 HOUR **MAKES:** 4 TO 6 SERVINGS

225 g/8 oz dry brown or French lentils
1 medium onion, chopped
150 g/5 oz chopped celery
150 g/5 oz diced carrots
1 tablespoon extra-virgin olive oil
1.1 litres/2 pints water
2 teaspoons instant chicken stock granules
2 cloves garlic, minced
½ teaspoon finely grated lemon peel
¼ teaspoon cayenne pepper
150 g/5 oz cubed cooked ham
85 g/3 oz chopped fresh spinach

1. Rinse and drain lentils; set aside.

2. In a large saucepan cook onion, celery, and carrots in hot oil about 10 minutes or until tender. Add lentils, the water, chicken stock granules, garlic, lemon peel, and black pepper. Bring to boiling; reduce heat. Cover and simmer for 45 minutes. Add ham; simmer, uncovered, for 15 minutes more. Stir in spinach. Serve immediately.

Nutrition Facts per serving: 261 cal., 7 g total fat (2 g sat. fat), 19 mg chol., 948 mg sodium, 36 g carbo., 17 g fibre, 20 g pro.

CHICKEN CHILLI

PREP: 25 MINUTES **COOK:** LOW 5 HOURS OR HIGH 2½ HOURS
MAKES: 4 SERVINGS

Non-stick olive oil cooking spray
450 g/1 lb skinless, boneless chicken breast halves, cut into 2.5-cm/1-inch pieces
2 400 g/14 oz cans cannellini beans (white kidney beans), rinsed and drained
565 ml/1 pint chicken stock
70 g/2½ oz chopped onion
85 g/3 oz chopped green pepper
1 small fresh jalapeño chilli, seeded and finely chopped*
½ teaspoon ground cumin
½ teaspoon dried oregano, crushed
¼ teaspoon ground white pepper
2 cloves garlic, minced
50 g/2 oz grated Monterey Jack or Cheddar cheese (optional)

1. Lightly coat a large frying-pan with non-stick cooking spray. Heat pan over medium-high heat. Brown chicken in hot pan; drain off fat.

2. In a 4 to 4.5-litre/7 to 8-pint slow cooker combine chicken, beans, stock, onion, pepper, chilli, cumin, oregano, white pepper, and garlic.

3. Cover and cook on low-heat setting for 5 to 6 hours or on high-heat setting for 2½ to 3 hours. If desired, sprinkle servings with cheese.

Nutrition Facts per serving: 275 cal., 2 g total fat (0 g sat. fat), 66 mg chol., 750 mg sodium, 33 g carbo., 11 g fibre, 40 g pro.

*Note: Because chillies contain oils that can burn your skin and eyes, wear rubber or plastic gloves when working with them. If your bare hands do touch the chillies, wash your hands well with soap and warm water.

CHICKEN SOUP WITH LIME

START TO FINISH: 30 MINUTES **MAKES:** 4 SERVINGS

340 g/12 oz skinless, boneless chicken breasts, cut into bite-size pieces
    Sea salt (optional)
    Freshly ground black pepper (optional)
  3 cloves garlic, minced
  1 tablespoon extra-virgin olive oil
  1 tablespoon hot chilli powder
  ½ teaspoon cumin seeds, crushed, or ¼ teaspoon ground cumin
  ¼ to ½ teaspoon crushed red pepper (optional)
850 ml/1½ pints chicken stock
  70 g/2½ oz chopped spring onions
  1 large tomato, chopped
  3 tablespoons lime juice
  1 tablespoon chopped fresh coriander

1. If desired, season chicken with sea salt and black pepper. In a large heavy casserole cook chicken and garlic in hot oil over medium-high heat until chicken is no longer pink. Stir in chilli powder, cumin, and, if desired, crushed red pepper. Cook and stir for 30 seconds. Stir in chicken stock and spring onions. Bring to boiling; reduce heat. Simmer, uncovered, for 10 minutes. Remove from heat. Stir in tomato, lime juice, and coriander.

Nutrition Facts per serving: 178 cal., 8 g total fat (1 g sat. fat), 45 mg chol., 719 mg sodium, 6 g carbo., 1 g fibre, 21 g pro.

FISH CHOWDER

PREP: 10 MINUTES **COOK:** 10 MINUTES **MAKES:** 4 TO 6 SERVINGS

450 g/1 lb fresh or frozen skinless, boneless sea bass, red snapper, and/or catfish fillets
70 g/2½ oz chopped onion
70 g/2½ oz bite-size fennel strips
2 cloves garlic, minced
1 tablespoon extra-virgin olive oil
850 ml/1½ pints water
2 fish stock cubes
1 tablespoon lemon juice
½ teaspoon instant chicken stock granules
½ teaspoon dried thyme, crushed
¼ teaspoon fennel seeds, crushed
Dash powdered saffron (optional)
1 bay leaf
4 tomatoes, halved lengthwise and thinly sliced
Lemon juice (optional)

1. Thaw fish, if frozen. Cut fish into 2-cm/¾-inch cubes. Rinse fish; pat dry with paper towels. Set aside.

2. In a large saucepan cook and stir onion, fennel strips, and garlic in hot oil over medium heat until tender. Stir in the water, fish stock cubes, the 1 tablespoon lemon juice, the chicken stock granules, thyme, fennel seeds, saffron (if desired), and bay leaf. Cook and stir until boiling.

3. Add fish and tomatoes. Return to boiling; reduce heat. Cover and simmer for 10 minutes. Discard bay leaf. If desired, stir in additional lemon juice to taste.

Nutrition Facts per serving: 176 cal., 6 g total fat (1 g sat. fat), 46 mg chol., 583 mg sodium, 8 g carbo., 2 g fibre, 22 g pro.

MINESTRONE

PREP: 30 MINUTES **COOK:** 30 MINUTES **MAKES:** 4 SERVINGS

  400 ml/14 fl oz chicken stock
    1 400 g/14 oz can tomatoes, cut up and undrained
  285 ml/½ pint water
  150 g/5 oz chopped onion
  115 g/4 oz shredded cabbage
  170 ml/6 fl oz tomato juice
    70 g/2½ oz chopped carrot
    70 g/2½ oz sliced celery
      1 tablespoon chopped fresh basil or 1 teaspoon dried basil, crushed
  ¼ teaspoon garlic powder
    1 400 g/14 oz can cannellini beans (white kidney beans), rinsed and drained
    1 medium courgette, sliced 0.5 cm/¼ inch thick
  125 g/4½ oz green beans
    50 g/2 oz whole wheat dried spaghetti or linguine, broken
      2 tablespoons finely grated Parmesan cheese

1. In a large heavy casserole combine stock, undrained tomatoes, the water, onion, cabbage, tomato juice, carrot, celery, basil, and garlic powder. Bring to boiling; reduce heat. Cover and simmer for 20 minutes.

2. Stir in cannellini beans, courgettes, green beans, and spaghetti. Return to boiling; reduce heat. Cover and simmer for 10 to 15 minutes more or until vegetables and pasta are tender. Sprinkle servings with Parmesan cheese.

Nutrition Facts per serving: 206 cal., 2 g total fat (1 g sat. fat), 3 mg chol.,
811 mg sodium, 43 g carbo., 10 g fibre, 13 g pro.

BEEF-BARLEY SOUP

PREP: 25 MINUTES **COOK:** 1¼ HOURS **MAKES:** 6 SERVINGS

340 g/12 oz beef or lamb stew meat, cut into 2.5-cm/1-inch cubes
1 tablespoon cooking oil
850 ml/1½ pints water
150 g/5 oz chopped onion
70 g/2½ oz chopped celery
90 g/3½ oz regular barley
2 teaspoons instant beef stock granules
1 teaspoon dried oregano or basil, crushed
¼ teaspoon freshly ground black pepper
2 cloves garlic, minced
1 bay leaf
225 g/8 oz frozen mixed vegetables
1 400 g/14 oz can diced tomatoes, undrained
170 g/6 oz parsnips cut into 1-cm/½-inch slices or peeled potatoes cut into
   1-cm/½-inch cubes

1. In a large saucepan brown meat in hot oil. Stir in the water, onion, celery, barley, beef granules, oregano, black pepper, garlic, and bay leaf. Bring to boiling; reduce heat. Cover and simmer for 1 hour for beef (45 minutes for lamb).

2. Stir in frozen vegetables, undrained tomatoes, and parsnips. Return to boiling; reduce heat. Cover and simmer about 15 minutes more or until meat and vegetables are tender. Discard bay leaf.

Nutrition Facts per serving: 210 cal., 6 g total fat (1 g sat. fat), 27 mg chol., 515 mg sodium, 23 g carbo., 4 g fibre, 16 g pro.

TOMATO-LENTIL SOUP

PREP: 20 MINUTES **COOK:** 45 MINUTES **MAKES:** 5 OR 6 SERVINGS

700 ml/1¼ pints water
1 400 g/14 oz can diced tomatoes, undrained
2 medium carrots, chopped
225 g/8 oz dry brown or French lentils, rinsed
150 g/5 oz chopped onion
70 g/2½ oz chopped celery
1 tablespoon instant chicken stock granules
2 cloves garlic, minced
1 bay leaf
½ teaspoon dried basil, crushed
½ teaspoon dried oregano, crushed
½ teaspoon dried thyme, crushed
150 g/5 oz regular brown rice
3 tablespoons chopped fresh flat-leaf parsley
½ teaspoon sea salt
½ teaspoon cider vinegar
¼ teaspoon freshly ground black pepper
Spring onions (optional)

1. In a large heavy casserole combine the water, undrained tomatoes, carrots, lentils, chopped onion, celery, chicken stock granules, garlic, bay leaf, basil, oregano, and thyme. Bring to boiling; reduce heat. Cover and simmer for 45 minutes.

2. Meanwhile, cook the brown rice according to the directions on the package.

3. Discard bay leaf. Stir parsley, sea salt, vinegar, and black pepper into lentil mixture. Stir in cooked rice. If desired, garnish with spring onions.

Nutrition Facts per serving: 283 cal., 1 g total fat (0 g sat. fat), 0 mg chol., 988 mg sodium, 53 g carbo., 15 g fibre, 14 g pro.

Tip: You can double the recipe. Seal, label, and freeze any remaining soup in a freezer container. To serve, let the soup thaw in the refrigerator overnight so you won't break up the lentils during heating. Reheat in a saucepan.

ROASTED ASPARAGUS PARMESAN

PREP: 10 MINUTES **BAKE:** 15 MINUTES **OVEN:** 200°C/400°F/GAS MARK 6 **MAKES:** 6 SERVINGS

> **900 g/2 lb fresh asparagus spears**
> **2 tablespoons extra-virgin olive oil**
> **Sea salt**
> **Freshly ground black pepper**
> **50 g/2 oz grated Parmesan cheese**

1. Snap off and discard woody base from asparagus spears. If desired, scrape off scales. Place asparagus in a 38×25×2.5-cm/15×10×1-inch baking pan. Drizzle with oil, tossing gently to coat. Spread out into a single layer. Sprinkle with sea salt and black pepper.

2. Bake in a 200°C/400°F/gas mark 6 oven about 15 minutes or until asparagus is crisp-tender, tossing asparagus occasionally. Transfer to a serving platter; sprinkle with Parmesan cheese.

Nutrition Facts per serving: 95 cal., 7 g total fat (2 g sat. fat), 8 mg chol., 102 mg sodium, 4 g carbo., 2 g fibre, 5 g pro.

BROCCOLI WITH LEMON AND DILL

START TO FINISH: 25 MINUTES **MAKES:** 6 TO 8 SERVINGS

70 g/2½ oz chopped onion or leek
1 clove garlic, minced
1 tablespoon extra-virgin olive oil
115 ml/4 fl oz chicken stock
675 g/1½ lb broccoli, cut into spears
1 tablespoon lemon juice
1 teaspoon cornflour
2 tablespoons chopped fresh dill or 1 teaspoon dried dill
Sea salt
Freshly ground black pepper
Lemon slices (optional)

1. In a large saucepan cook and stir onion and garlic in hot oil about 3 minutes or until tender. Add stock; bring to boiling. Add broccoli. Return to boiling; reduce heat. Cover and simmer for 8 to 10 minutes or until tender. Transfer vegetables to a serving platter, reserving stock in pan (add additional stock, if necessary, to measure 115 ml/4 fl oz).

2. In a small bowl combine lemon juice and cornflour; add to stock in saucepan. Cook and stir until thickened and bubbly; cook and stir for 2 minutes more. Stir in dill. Season to taste with sea salt and black pepper. Spoon sauce over vegetables; toss to coat. If desired, garnish with lemon slices.

Nutrition Facts per serving: 55 cal., 3 g total fat (0 g sat. fat), 0 mg chol., 90 mg sodium, 7 g carbo., 2 g fibre, 2 g pro.

COURGETTES AND PEPPERS WITH FETA

START TO FINISH: 25 MINUTES **MAKES:** 6 SERVINGS

1 tablespoon extra-virgin olive oil
150 g/5 oz chopped onion
3 medium courgettes, sliced 0.5 cm/¼ inch thick
2 tablespoons water
½ teaspoon ground cumin
½ of a 200 g/7 oz jar roasted red peppers, drained and cut into strips
2 tablespoons chopped fresh basil
Sea salt
Freshly ground black pepper
2 tablespoons crumbled feta cheese

1. In a large frying-pan heat oil over medium heat. Add onion; cook and stir about 5 minutes or until tender. Add courgettes, the water, and cumin to pan; reduce heat. Cover and simmer for 3 to 5 minutes or until courgettes are crisp-tender.

2. Stir roasted pepper strips and basil into courgette mixture; heat through. Season to taste with sea salt and black pepper. Sprinkle with feta cheese.

Nutrition Facts per serving: 56 cal., 3 g total fat (1 g sat. fat), 2 mg chol., 108 mg sodium, 6 g carbo., 2 g fibre, 2 g pro.

WILTED SPINACH WITH WALNUTS AND BLUE CHEESE

START TO FINISH: 15 MINUTES **MAKES:** 4 SERVINGS

225 g/8 oz fresh spinach or Swiss chard leaves
2 teaspoons extra-virgin olive oil
2 tablespoons chopped walnuts, toasted
1 tablespoon crumbled blue cheese (such as Gorgonzola, Stilton, or Danish blue)
¼ teaspoon coarsely ground black pepper

1. Cut spinach into 2.5-cm/1-inch-wide strips. In a large frying-pan heat oil over medium-high heat. Add spinach. Cook and stir, uncovered, about 1 minute or just until wilted. Remove from heat.

2. Divide spinach among 4 serving bowls. Top with walnuts and crumbled blue cheese; sprinkle with black pepper.

Nutrition Facts per serving: 65 cal., 6 g total fat (1 g sat. fat), 2 mg chol., 74 mg sodium, 2 g carbo., 2 g fibre, 3 g pro.

PESTO GREEN BEANS AND TOMATOES

PREP: 20 MINUTES **COOK:** 10 MINUTES **MAKES:** 6 TO 8 SERVINGS

675 g/1½ lb fresh green beans, trimmed
225 g/8 oz small tomatoes (yellow, red, and/or orange), halved
  50 ml/2 fl oz Pesto Vinaigrette
    Sea salt
    Freshly ground black pepper

1. In a covered large saucepan cook beans in a small amount of boiling salted water for 10 to 15 minutes or until crisp-tender. Drain and rinse under cold water. Drain and pat dry with paper towels.

2. In a large bowl toss green beans and tomatoes with Pesto Vinaigrette. Add more vinaigrette, if necessary. Season to taste with sea salt and black pepper. Serve immediately or chill in the refrigerator for up to 8 hours.

Pesto Vinaigrette: In a medium bowl combine 85 g/3 oz bought basil pesto, 3 tablespoons white wine vinegar, and 1 tablespoon lemon juice. Add 50 ml/2 fl oz extra-virgin olive oil in a thin, steady stream, whisking constantly until combined. Add sea salt and ground white pepper to taste. Refrigerate until ready to use or for up to 3 days.
Nutrition Facts per serving: 128 cal., 8 g total fat (1 g sat. fat), 1 mg chol., 275 mg sodium, 13 g carbo., 5 g fibre, 4 g pro.

STEAMED RED CHARD

START TO FINISH: 45 MINUTES **MAKES:** 6 SERVINGS

1.4 kg/3 lb red Swiss chard, stems removed and leaves cut crosswise into
    1-cm/½-inch strips
2 large onions, chopped
2 tablespoons extra-virgin olive oil
2 cloves garlic, minced
50 ml/2 fl oz sherry vinegar or red wine vinegar
½ teaspoon sea salt
½ teaspoon freshly ground black pepper

1. Fill 4.5-litre/8-pint heavy casserole with water to a depth of 2.5 cm/1 inch. Bring water to boiling. Place a steamer basket in the casserole. Place one-third of the Swiss chard in the steamer basket. Cover and steam about 5 minutes or until chard is tender. Remove wilted chard from steamer basket and place in a large colander placed over a large bowl to drain; set aside. Repeat with remaining chard.

2. In the same casserole cook onions in hot oil over medium heat until tender. Add garlic; cook for 10 seconds. Add steamed chard, vinegar, sea salt, and black pepper. Cook and stir until heated through.

Nutrition Facts per serving: 76 cal., 4 g total fat (1 g sat. fat), 0 mg chol., 463 mg sodium, 10 g carbo., 3 g fibre, 3 g pro.

SWEET PEPPER DIP

PREP: 25 MINUTES **GRILL:** 10 MINUTES **STAND:** 10 MINUTES
CHILL: 1 TO 24 HOURS **MAKES:** 450 G/1 LB

**2 large red peppers, quartered lengthwise
4 teaspoons extra-virgin olive oil
1 225 g/8 oz carton low-fat soured cream
1 85 g/3 oz package low-fat cream cheese, softened
1 tablespoon extra-virgin olive oil (optional)
½ teaspoon sea salt
2 tablespoons finely chopped spring onion
2 tablespoons chopped fresh basil or 1 teaspoon dried basil, crushed
Assorted vegetable dippers, crackers, and/or crisps (optional)**

1. Brush pepper pieces with the 4 teaspoons olive oil. Place peppers, cut sides up, on the rack of grill a barbecue and grill about 10 minutes or until pepper skins are blistered and dark.

2. Wrap pepper pieces tightly in foil and let stand for 10 to 15 minutes or until cool enough to handle. Unwrap peppers. Using a paring knife, gently pull the skin off pepper pieces.

3. In a blender or food processor combine grilled peppers, soured cream, cream cheese, the 1 tablespoon olive oil (if desired), and the sea salt. Cover and blend or process until smooth. Transfer to a medium bowl. Stir in spring onion and basil. Cover and chill for 1 to 24 hours. If desired, serve dip with vegetable dippers, crackers, and/or crisps.

Nutrition Facts per 2 tablespoons dip: 42 cal., 3 g total fat (1 g sat. fat), 8 mg chol., 81 mg sodium, 2 g carbo., 0 g fibre, 1 g pro.

APPLE AND PEPPER SLAW

PREP: 20 MINUTES **STAND:** 20 MINUTES **MAKES:** 3 OR 4 SIDE-DISH SERVINGS

115 g/8 oz shredded red and/or green cabbage
1 small red or green pepper, cut into thin strips
50 g/2 oz chopped apple
70 g/2½ oz chopped carrot
40 g/1½ oz thinly sliced celery
Sea salt
85 g/3 fl oz plain low-fat yogurt
About 1 teaspoon bought ranch salad dressing
2 tablespoons chopped fresh chives

1. In a large colander combine cabbage, peppers, apple, carrot, and celery. Sprinkle with a little sea salt; let stand for 20 minutes. Drain off any liquid. Transfer cabbage mixture to a large serving bowl.

2. For dressing, in a small bowl stir together yogurt, ranch dressing, and chives. If necessary, stir in a little water to make desired consistency.

3. Pour dressing over cabbage mixture. Toss to coat. Serve immediately.

Nutrition Facts per serving: 100 cal., 1 g total fat (0 g sat. fat), 2 mg chol.,
301 mg sodium, 13 g carbo., 3 g fibre, 3 g pro.

CABBAGE SALAD WITH ASIAN-STYLE VINAIGRETTE

START TO FINISH: 35 MINUTES **MAKES:** 4 SERVINGS

115 g/4 oz mangetout peas, trimmed
170 g/6 oz shredded Chinese leaves
50 g/2 oz fresh bean sprouts
150 g/5 oz bite-size red pepper strips
70 g/2½ oz thinly sliced spring onions
50 g/2 oz shelled fresh or frozen sweet soya beans (edamame), thawed
3 tablespoons chopped fresh coriander
1 teaspoon grated fresh ginger
2 cloves garlic, minced
1 recipe Asian-Style Vinaigrette (see recipe, page 155)
Sea salt
Freshly ground black pepper

1. In a covered medium saucepan cook mangetout peas in a small amount of boiling water for 1 minute. Drain. Submerse in ice water to cool quickly; drain.

2. In a large bowl combine mangetout peas, Chinese leaves, bean sprouts, pepper strips, spring onions, soya beans, coriander, ginger, and garlic. Add Asian Vinaigrette; toss well. Season to taste with sea salt and black pepper.

Nutrition Facts per serving: 135 cal., 5 g total fat (1 g sat. fat), 0 mg chol., 1,079 mg sodium, 17 g carbo., 4 g fibre, 10 g pro.

SPINACH-APRICOT SALAD

START TO FINISH: 20 MINUTES **MAKES:** 4 SERVINGS

340 g/12 oz torn fresh baby spinach leaves
50 g/2 oz dried apricots, snipped
1 tablespoon extra-virgin olive oil
1 clove garlic, thinly sliced or minced
4 teaspoons balsamic vinegar
Sea salt
Freshly ground black pepper
2 tablespoons slivered almonds, toasted

1. If desired, remove stems from spinach. In a large bowl combine spinach and apricots; set aside.

2. In a 30-cm/12-inch frying-pan heat oil over medium heat. Add garlic; cook and stir until golden. Stir in balsamic vinegar. Bring to boiling; remove from heat.

3. Add spinach mixture to vinegar mixture. Return to heat. Toss mixture in frying-pan for about 1 minute or just until spinach is wilted.

4. Transfer spinach mixture to a serving dish. Season to taste with sea salt and black pepper. Sprinkle with almonds. Serve immediately.

Nutrition Facts per serving: 95 cal., 6 g total fat (1 g sat. fat), 0 mg chol., 113 mg sodium, 9 g carbo., 7 g fibre, 3 g pro.

MARINATED COURGETTES AND MUSHROOMS

PREP: 25 MINUTES **STAND:** 10 MINUTES **MARINATE:** 8 TO 24 HOURS **MAKES:** 6 TO 8 SERVINGS

> 2 tablespoons lemon juice
> 1 tablespoon chopped shallot
> 1 clove garlic, minced
> ⅛ teaspoon sea salt
> 1 small courgette
> 1 small yellow pattypan squash
> 115 g/4 oz small whole fresh mushrooms
> ½ of a small red pepper, cut into squares
> 1 tablespoon extra-virgin olive oil
> ¾ teaspoon chopped fresh tarragon or oregano or ⅛ teaspoon dried tarragon or oregano, crushed
> ⅛ teaspoon freshly ground black pepper

1. In a small bowl combine lemon juice, shallot, garlic, and sea salt. Let stand for 10 minutes. Meanwhile, using a vegetable peeler, shave off long, thin strips of courgette and pattypan squash. In a self-sealing plastic bag set in a large bowl combine courgettes, pattypan squash, mushrooms, and pepper.

2. Whisk oil, tarragon, and black pepper into lemon juice mixture. Pour marinade over vegetables in bag. Seal bag; turn to coat vegetables. Marinate in the refrigerator for 8 to 24 hours, turning bag occasionally.

3. To serve, drain vegetables, reserving marinade. Arrange vegetables on serving plates or a serving platter; drizzle with reserved marinade.

Nutrition Facts per serving: 38 cal., 3 g total fat (0 g sat. fat), 0 mg chol., 44 mg sodium, 3 g carbo., 1 g fibre, 1 g pro.

ASPARAGUS AND BARLEY PILAF

START TO FINISH: 50 MINUTES **MAKES:** 3 MAIN-DISH
OR 6 SIDE-DISH SERVINGS

200 g/7 oz regular barley
2 tablespoons extra-virgin olive oil
70 g/2½ oz finely chopped onion
1 clove garlic, minced
400 ml/14 fl oz chicken or vegetable stock
225 g/8 oz fresh asparagus, cut into 2.5 cm/1-inch pieces
70 g/2½ oz shredded carrot
25 g/1 oz finely grated Parmesan cheese
3 tablespoons chopped fresh basil
    Sea salt
    Freshly ground black pepper

1. In a large saucepan cook barley in 1 tablespoon of the oil over medium heat about 5 minutes or until lightly toasted, stirring often. Add onion, garlic, and remaining 1 tablespoon oil; cook until onion is tender.

2. In a small saucepan heat stock. Slowly add 170 ml/6 fl oz of the stock to barley mixture, stirring constantly. Continue to cook and stir over medium heat until liquid is absorbed. Add another 115 ml/4 fl oz of the stock, stirring constantly. Continue to cook and stir until the liquid is absorbed. Add another 115 ml/4 fl oz of the stock; cook and stir until liquid is almost all absorbed.

3. Add asparagus and carrot; continue cooking until all the liquid is absorbed and the barley is tender. (This should take about 30 minutes total.)

4. Remove from heat. Stir in cheese and basil; season to taste with sea salt and black pepper.

Nutrition Facts per main-dish serving: 166 cal., 7 g total fat (2 g sat. fat), 6 mg chol., 349 mg sodium, 22 g carbo., 4 g fibre, 5 g pro.

GRAIN MEDLEY WITH ASIAN SEASONINGS

PREP: 20 MINUTES **COOK:** 30 TO 60 MINUTES (DEPENDS ON GRAINS USED) **STAND:** 5 MINUTES **MAKES:** 8 SERVINGS

- 2 stalks celery, cut into 2.5-cm/1-inch pieces
- 1 large carrot, cut into 2.5-cm/1-inch pieces
- 1 small onion, cut into 2.5-cm/1-inch pieces
- 2 tablespoons Chinese black bean sauce
- 1 5-cm/2-inch piece fresh ginger, sliced
- 2 cloves garlic, halved
- 225 g/8 oz mixed grains* (such as spelt; brown rice; wild rice; brown, French, or green lentils; regular barley; and/or quinoa), rinsed and drained
- 700 ml/1¼ pints water
- ¼ teaspoon sea salt
- ¼ teaspoon freshly ground black pepper

1. Cut a 30-cm/12-inch square from a double thickness of 100% cotton cheesecloth. Place celery, carrot, onion, black bean sauce, ginger, and garlic in centre of the cheesecloth square. Bring up corners and tie with 100% cotton string.

2. In a 2.2 to 3.5-litre/4 to 6-pint saucepan combine desired grains, the water, and cheesecloth bag. Bring to boiling; reduce heat. Cover and simmer for 30 to 60 minutes or until grains are tender. Remove from heat. Let stand, covered, for 5 minutes. Discard cheesecloth bag, allowing any liquid to drain off. Drain any excess liquid from grains. Stir in sea salt and black pepper.

Nutrition Facts per serving: 110 cal., 1 g total fat (0 g sat. fat), 0 mg chol., 153 mg sodium, 21 g carbo., 4 g fibre, 5 g pro.

*Note: You can cook spelt, brown rice, and wild rice together; they will take 45 to 60 minutes to cook. You can cook lentils, barley, and quinoa together; they will take about 30 minutes to cook. If you want to combine shorter-cooking grains with longer-cooking grains, cook the longer-cooking grains for 20 to 30 minutes and then add the shorter-cooking grains and cook about 30 minutes more or until tender.

GRAIN MEDLEY WITH MEDITERRANEAN SEASONINGS

PREP: 20 MINUTES **COOK:** 30 TO 60 MINUTES (DEPENDS ON GRAINS USED) **STAND:** 5 MINUTES **MAKES:** 8 SERVINGS

  2 stalks celery, cut into 2.5-cm/1-inch pieces
  1 large carrot, cut into 2.5-cm/1-inch pieces
  1 small onion, cut into 2.5-cm/1-inch pieces
  2 bay leaves
 10 fresh thyme sprigs
 10 fresh flat-leaf parsley sprigs
225 g/8 oz mixed grains* (such as spelt; brown rice; wild rice; brown, French, or
    green lentils; regular barley; and/or quinoa), rinsed and drained
700 ml/1¼ pints water
  ¼ teaspoon sea salt
  ¼ teaspoon freshly ground black pepper

1. Cut a 30-cm/12-inch square from a double thickness of 100% cotton cheesecloth. Place celery, carrot, onion, bay leaves, thyme, and parsley in centre of the cheesecloth square. Bring up corners and tie with 100% cotton string.

2. In a 2 to 3.5-litre/4 to 6-pint saucepan combine desired grains, the water, and cheesecloth bag. Bring to boiling; reduce heat. Cover and simmer for 30 to 60 minutes or until grains are tender. Remove from heat. Let stand, covered, for 5 minutes. Discard cheesecloth bag, allowing any liquid to drain off. Drain any excess liquid from grains. Stir in sea salt and black pepper.

Nutrition Facts per serving: 103 cal., 1 g total fat (0 g sat. fat), 0 mg chol., 64 mg sodium, 20 g carbo., 4 g fibre, 4 g pro.

*Note: You can cook spelt, brown rice, and wild rice together; they will take 45 to 60 minutes to cook. You can cook lentils, barley, and quinoa together; they will take about 30 minutes to cook. If you want to combine shorter-cooking grains with longer-cooking grains, cook the longer-cooking grains for 20 to 30 minutes and then add the shorter-cooking grains and cook about 30 minutes more or until tender.

GRAIN MEDLEY WITH MEXICAN SEASONINGS

PREP: 20 MINUTES **COOK:** 30 TO 60 MINUTES (DEPENDS ON GRAINS USED) **STAND:** 5 MINUTES **MAKES:** 8 SERVINGS

2 stalks celery, cut into 2.5-cm/1-inch pieces
1 large carrot, cut into 2.5-cm/1-inch pieces
1 small onion, cut into 2.5-cm/1-inch pieces
3 cloves garlic, halved
3 canned chipotle chillies in adobo sauce plus 1 tablespoon adobo sauce
4 sprigs fresh Mexican oregano or regular oregano
225 g/8 oz mixed grains* (such as spelt; brown rice; wild rice; brown, French, or green lentils; regular barley; and/or quinoa), rinsed and drained
700 ml/1¼ pints water
¼ teaspoon sea salt
¼ teaspoon freshly ground black pepper

1. Cut a 30-cm/12-inch square from a double thickness of 100% cotton cheesecloth. Place celery, carrot, onion, garlic, chipotle peppers and sauce, and oregano in the centre of the cheesecloth square. Bring up corners and tie with 100% cotton string.

2. In a 2 to 3.5-litre/4 to 6-pint saucepan combine desired grains, the water, and cheesecloth bag. Bring to boiling; reduce heat. Cover and simmer for 30 to 60 minutes or until grains are tender. Remove from heat. Let stand, covered, for 5 minutes. Discard cheesecloth bag, allowing any liquid to drain off. Drain any excess liquid from grains. Stir in sea salt and black pepper.

Nutrition Facts per serving: 103 cal., 1 g total fat (0 g sat. fat), 0 mg chol., 73 mg sodium, 20 g carbo., 4 g fibre, 4 g pro.

*Note: You can cook spelt, brown rice, and wild rice together; they will take 45 to 60 minutes to cook. You can cook lentils, barley, and quinoa together; they will take about 30 minutes to cook. If you want to combine shorter-cooking grains with longer-cooking grains, cook the longer-cooking grains for 20 to 30 minutes and then add the shorter-cooking grains and cook about 30 minutes more or until tender.

WHEAT BERRY TABBOULEH

PREP: 25 MINUTES **COOK:** 1 HOUR (WHEAT BERRIES)
MAKES: 6 SERVINGS

  200 g/7 oz wheat berries, cooked*
  85 g/3 oz chopped tomato
  85 g/3 oz chopped cucumber
  6 tablespoons chopped fresh flat-leaf parsley
  40 g/1½ oz thinly sliced spring onions
  1 tablespoon chopped fresh mint
  3 tablespoons extra-virgin olive oil
  3 tablespoons lemon juice
  ¼ teaspoon sea salt
    Sliced cucumber (optional)
    Sliced lemon (optional)

1. In a large bowl combine cooked wheat berries, tomato, chopped cucumber, parsley, spring onions, and mint.

2. For dressing, in a screw-top jar combine oil, lemon juice, and sea salt. Cover and shake well. Drizzle dressing over wheat berry mixture; toss to coat.

3. To serve, if desired, arrange sliced cucumber and lemon around edge of bowl.

Nutrition Facts per serving: 142 cal., 7 g total fat (1 g sat. fat), 0 mg chol., 86 mg sodium, 17 g carbo., 2 g fibre, 3 g pro.

Make-ahead directions: Prepare as above through step 2. Cover and chill for up to 24 hours. To serve, if desired, arrange sliced cucumber and lemon around edge of bowl.

*Note: To cook wheat berries, in a medium saucepan bring 450 ml/¾ pint vegetable or chicken stock to boiling. Add 200 g/7 oz rinsed and drained wheat berries. Return to boiling; reduce heat. Cover and simmer about 1 hour or until tender; drain. Cover and refrigerate for up to 3 days.

WHEAT BERRY AND LENTIL SALAD

PREP: 30 MINUTES **COOK:** 1½ HOURS **MAKES:** 12 SERVINGS

700 ml/1¼ pints water
90 g/3½ oz wheat berries, rinsed and drained
115 g/4 oz brown or French lentils, rinsed and drained
85 ml/3 fl oz lemon juice
2 tablespoons finely chopped shallots
1 clove garlic, minced
1 tablespoon Dijon-style mustard
85 g/3 fl oz extra-virgin olive oil
½ teaspoon crushed red pepper
Sea salt
Freshly ground black pepper
1 400 g/14 oz can chickpeas, rinsed and drained
1 medium tomato, chopped
1 small cucumber, chopped
6 tablespoons chopped fresh flat-leaf parsley
70 g/2½ oz sliced spring onions
2 tablespoons torn fresh basil leaves or 2 teaspoons dried basil, crushed

1. In a medium saucepan combine the water and wheat berries. Bring to boiling; reduce heat. Cover and simmer for 1 hour. Stir in lentils; continue to cook about 30 minutes more or until lentils and wheat berries are tender. Drain, discarding cooking liquid. Cool to room temperature.

2. For dressing, in a medium bowl combine lemon juice, shallots, and garlic. Let stand for 5 minutes. Whisk in mustard. Add oil in a thin, steady stream, whisking constantly until combined. Stir in crushed red pepper. Season to taste with sea salt and black pepper. Set aside.

3. In a large bowl combine cooked wheat berries and lentils, chickpeas, tomato, cucumber, parsley, spring onions, and basil. Add dressing; toss to coat. Season to taste with sea salt and black pepper.

Nutrition Facts per serving: 162 cal., 7 g total fat (1 g sat. fat), 0 mg chol., 202 mg sodium, 22 g carbo., 5 g fibre, 6 g pro.

STRAWBERRY-CITRUS SLUSH

START TO FINISH: 10 MINUTES **MAKES:** 3 SERVINGS

170 g/6 oz frozen unsweetened whole strawberries
1 340 ml/12 fl oz can low-calorie grapefruit carbonated beverage
Handful ice cubes
2 teaspoons sugar substitute (Splenda®)
¼ teaspoon orange extract or lime extract (optional)

1. In a blender combine strawberries, carbonated beverage, ice cubes, sugar substitute, and, if desired, orange extract. Cover and blend until smooth. Divide slush evenly among 3 wine glasses.

Nutrition Facts per serving: 22 cal., 0 g total fat (0 g sat. fat), 0 mg chol., 24 mg sodium, 6 g carbo., 1 g fibre, 0 g pro.

SUMMER BERRIES WITH ALMOND SAUCE

START TO FINISH: 10 MINUTES **MAKES:** 6 SERVINGS

225 g/8 oz fresh blackberries
115 g/4 oz fresh raspberries
170 ml/6 fl oz low-fat soured cream or plain low-fat yogurt
    Sugar substitute (Splenda®) to equal 1½ teaspoons sugar
½ to ¾ teaspoon almond extract

1. Divide blackberries and raspberries evenly among 6 dessert dishes. Set aside.

2. In a small bowl combine soured cream, sugar substitute, and almond extract. Spoon mixture evenly over berries.

Nutrition Facts per serving: 69 cal., 3 g total fat (2 g sat. fat), 10 mg chol., 21 mg sodium, 8 g carbo., 4 g fibre, 3 g pro.

TROPICAL FRUIT POPS

PREP: 15 MINUTES **FREEZE:** 6 HOURS **MAKES:** 8 LARGE OR
12 SMALL POPS

> **115 ml/4 fl oz boiling water**
> **1 package sugar-free lemon-, mixed fruit-, or strawberry-flavour jelly**
> **1 400 g/14 oz can crushed pineapple**
> **2 medium bananas, cut into chunks**

1. Stir together the boiling water and the jelly until jelly dissolves. Pour into a blender. Add undrained pineapple and banana chunks. Cover and blend until smooth.

2. Pour a scant 50 g/2 oz of the fruit mixture into each of eight 150 to 170 g/5 to 6 oz paper or plastic drink cups. (Or pour a scant 35 g/1¼ oz into each of twelve 85 g/3 oz cups. Cover each cup with foil. Using the tip of a knife, make a small hole in the foil over each cup. Insert a wooden stick into the cup through the hole. Freeze about 6 hours or until firm.

3. To serve, quickly dip the cups in warm water to slightly soften fruit mixture. Remove foil and loosen sides of pops from drink cups. Tear off the paper.

Nutrition Facts per large pop: 65 cal., 0 g total fat (0 g sat. fat), 0 mg chol., 29 mg sodium, 15 g carbo., 1 g fibre, 1 g pro.

APPLE-BLUEBERRY TARTS

PREP: 30 MINUTES **BAKE:** 40 MINUTES **COOL:** 15 MINUTES
OVEN: 190°C/375°F/GAS MARK 5 **MAKES:** 6 TARTS

  2 medium cooking apples, peeled, cored, and chopped
85 g/3 oz fresh or frozen blueberries
  1 tablespoon sugar substitute (Splenda®)
    or 2 tablespoons honey
¼ teaspoon ground allspice
200 g/7 oz whole wheat pastry flour
  ¼ teaspoon sea salt
  ⅛ teaspoon ground allspice
85 ml/3 fl oz extra-virgin olive oil
  3 tablespoons fat-free milk

1. In a medium bowl combine apples, blueberries, sugar substitute, and the ¼ teaspoon allspice; set aside.

2. In another medium bowl stir together whole wheat pastry flour, sea salt, and the ⅛ teaspoon allspice. Add oil and milk all at once to flour mixture. Stir lightly with a fork until dough comes together. Divide dough into 6 portions. Using six 9- to 10-cm/3½- to 4-inch individual tart pans with removable bottoms, press one dough portion on the bottom and up the side of each tart pan. Divide fruit mixture among pastry-lined pans. Place tart pans on a large baking sheet. Place a large piece of foil over tart pans; press down lightly around the edges to seal.

3. Bake in a 190°C/375°F/gas mark 5 oven for 20 minutes; remove foil. Bake about 20 minutes more or until fruit is tender. Let cool in tart pans on a wire rack for 15 minutes. Carefully remove sides of tart pans. Serve warm or cool.

Nutrition Facts per tart: 205 cal., 12 g total fat (1 g sat. fat), 0 mg chol., 84 mg sodium, 23 g carbo., 3 g fibre, 3 g pro.

PEACHY BERRY COBBLER

PREP: 35 MINUTES **BAKE:** 15 MINUTES **OVEN:** 200°C/400°F/GAS MARK 6 **MAKES:** 8 SERVINGS

150 g/5 oz whole wheat pastry flour
1½ teaspoons baking powder
¼ teaspoon ground ginger or ground cinnamon
⅛ teaspoon sea salt
2 tablespoons butter
85 ml/3 fl oz cold water
4 teaspoons cornflour
2 tablespoons sugar substitute (Splenda®)
    or 2 tablespoons honey
450 g/1 lb fresh or frozen peeled, unsweetened peach slices
225 g/8 oz fresh or frozen unsweetened raspberries and/or blueberries
85 ml/3 fl oz plain fat-free yogurt
1 slightly beaten egg
Ground ginger or ground cinnamon (optional)

1. For topping, in a medium bowl stir together whole wheat pastry flour, baking powder, the ¼ teaspoon ginger, and the sea salt. Using a pastry blender, cut in butter until mixture resembles coarse crumbs. Set aside.

2. For filling, in a large saucepan stir together the water and cornflour until combined. Stir in sugar substitute. Add peach slices. Cook and stir until thickened and bubbly. Stir in raspberries and/or blueberries. Cook, stirring gently, until bubbly. Cover and keep filling hot while finishing topping.

3. To finish topping, in a small bowl stir together yogurt and egg. Add yogurt mixture to flour mixture, stirring just until moistened.

4. Divide filling among eight 170 g/6 oz custard cups or four 275 to 340 g/10 to 12 oz baking dishes.* Drop the topping from a spoon onto hot filling. Drop 1 mound into each custard cup or 2 mounds into each dish. Place custard cups or baking dishes on a baking sheet.

5. Bake in a 200°C/400°F/gas mark 6 oven for 15 to 20 minutes or until a toothpick inserted into topping comes out clean. Cool slightly. If desired, sprinkle with additional ginger. Serve warm.

Nutrition Facts per serving: 128 cal., 4 g total fat (2 g sat. fat), 35 mg chol., 114 mg sodium, 22 g carbo., 4 g fibre, 4 g pro.

*Note: To make one large cobbler, transfer hot filling to a 2.2-litre/4-pint square baking dish. Drop topping from a spoon into 8 mounds on top of hot filling. Bake in a 200°C/400°F/gas mark 6 oven about 20 minutes or until a toothpick inserted into topping comes out clean.

REFERENCES

Welcome to Your New Lifestyle

Trichopoulou A, et al. Cancer and Mediterranean dietary traditions. *Cancer Epidemiol Biomarkers Prev* 2000; 9:869-73.

Triochopoulou A. Mediterranean diet and longevity. *Br J Nutr* 2000 Dec; 84(Supp 2): S205-9.

Keys A. Seven countries: A multivariate analysis of death and coronary heart disease. Cambridge, MA. Harvard University Press, 1980.

Lampe J. Health effects of vegetables and fruits: assessing mechanisms of action in human experimental studies. *Am J Clin Nutr* 1999; 70, 475-490.

Trichopoulou A, et al. Modified Mediterranean diet and survival: EPIC elderly prospective cohort study. *BMJ* Apr/2005; 330(7498):991.

Trichopoulou A, Costacou T, Bamia C, Trichopoulou D. Adherence to a Mediterranean diet and survival in a Greek population. *N Engl J Med* 2003; 348(26):2599-608.

What Is the Sonoma Diet?

Joshipura KJ, Hu FB, et al. The effect of fruit and vegetable intake on risk for coronary heart disease. *Annals of Internal Medicine* 2001; 134:1106-1114.

Steinmetz KA, Potter JD. Vegetables, fruit, and cancer prevention. *J Am Diet Assoc* 1996; 96:1027-1039.

Etherton P, et al. High monounsaturated fatty acid diets lower both plasma cholesterol and triacylglycerol concentrations. *Am J Clin Nutr* 1999; 70, 1009-15.

Mckeown et al. Whole grain intake is favorable associated with metabolic risk factors for type 2 diabetes and cardiovascular disease. *Am J Clin Nutr* 2002; 76:390-98.

Drewnoski and Carneros. Bitter taste, phytonutrients, and the consumer: A review. *Am J Clin Nutr* 2000; 72:1424-35.

Zelman K and Kennedy E. Naturally nutrient rich … putting more power on Americans' plates. *Nutrition Today* 2005; 40:2.

Howarth NC, Saltzman E, Roberts SB. Dietary fiber and weight regulation. *Nutr Rev* 2001; 59:129-139.

Mattes R, et al. Appetite: Measurement and manipulation misgivings. *J AM Diet Assoc* 2005; 105:S87-S97.

Weigle D, et al. A high-protein diet induces sustained reductions in appetite, ad libitum caloric intake, and body weight despite compensatory changes in diurnal plasma leptin and ghrelin concentrations. *Am J Clin Nutr* 2005; 82(1):41-8.

The Insulin Resistance Atherosclerosis Study, *AM J Clin Nutr* 2003.

Salmeron J, Manson J, Stampfer M, et al. Dietary fiber, glycemic load, and risk of non insulin-dependent diabetes mellitus in women. *JAMA* 1997; 277:472-77.

Slavin J, Jacobs D, Marquart L. Whole grain consumption and chronic disease: protective mechanisms. *Nutr Cancer* 1997; 27:14-21.

Bruinsma K, Taren D. Dieting, essential fatty acid intake and depression. *Nutrition Reviews* 2000; 58:98-108.

Wells AS, Read NW, Laugharne JDE, Ahlumalia NS. Alterations in mood after changing to a low-fat diet. *Br J Nutr* 1998; 79:23-30.

Locke C and Stoll A. Omega-3 fatty acids in major depression. *World Review Nutr Diet* 2001; 89:173-185.

Dallman M, Pecoraro N, et al. Chronic stress and obesity: A new view of comfort food. *PNAS* Sept 30, 2003; 100, 20:11696-11701.

Katan, Grundy, Willett. Should a low fat, high-carbohydrate diet be recommended for everyone? Beyond low fat diets. *N Eng J Med* 1997; 337:563-567.

Denke M. Metabolic effects of high-protein, low-carbohydrate diets. *AM J Cardiol* 2001; 88:59-61.

Tapper-Gardzina Y, Cotugna N et al. Should you recommend a low-carb, high-protein diet? *Nurse Prac* 2002; 27:52-57.

The Top Ten Sonoma Diet Power Foods

Willet WC. Diet and health: What should we eat? *Science* 1994; 532-7.

Joshipura KJ, Hu FB, et al. The effect of fruit and vegetable intake on risk for coronary heart disease. *Annals of Internal Medicine* 2001; 134:1106-1114.

Am J Clin Nutr 2000; 72:922-8.

Steinmetz KA, Potter JD. Vegetables, fruit, and cancer prevention. *J Am Diet Assoc* 1996; 96:1027-1039.

Rice-Evans CA, Miller NJ, Bolwell PG, Bramely PM, Pridham JB. The relative antioxidant activities of plant derived polyphenolic flavonoids. *Free Radic Res* 1995; 22:375-83.

Wise JA, Morein, RJ, Sanderson R, Blum K. Changes in plasma carotenoid, alpha tocopherol, and lipid peroxide levels in response to supplementation with concentrated fruit and vegetable extracts; a pilot study. *Curr Ther Res Clin Exp* 1996; 57:445-61

Kivipelto M, et al. Body mass index, clustering of vascular risk factors, risk of dementia: A longitudinal population based study. *Neurol Bio of Aging*. Elsevior: Vol 25 (Supp 2), 2004.

Kang J, et al. Fruit and vegetable consumption and cognitive decline in women. *Neurol Bio of Aging*. Elsevior: Vol 25 (Supp 2), 2004.

Eichholzer M, Luthy J, Gutzwiller F, Stahelin H. The role of folate, antioxidant vitamins and other constituents in fruit and vegetables in the prevention of cardiovascular disease: The epidemiological evidence. *Int J Vitam Nutr Res* 2001; 71(1):5-17.

Hemila H. Vitamin C intake and susceptibility to the common cold. *British Journal of Nutrition* 1997; 77, 59-72.

Almonds: A nutrition and health perspective. Modesto, California: Almond Board of California, 2003.

Fulgoni V. Almonds lower blood cholesterol and LDL-cholesterol but not HDL-cholesterol or triglycerides in human subjects: Results of a meta-analysis. Presented at Experimental Biology, 2002.

Jenkins DJ, Kendall CW, Marchie A, Parker TL, Connelly PW, Quian W, Haight JS, Faulkner D, Vidgen E, Lapsley KG, and Spiller GA. Dose response of almonds on coronary heart disease risk factors: Blood lipids, oxidized low-density lipoproteins, lipoprotein (a), homocysteine, and pulmonary nitric oxide: A randomized, controlled, crossover trial. *Circulation* 2002; 106(11):1327-1332.

Lovejoy JC, Most MM, Lefevre M, Greenway FL, and Rood JC. Effects of diets enriched in almonds on insulin action and serum lipids in adults with normal glucose tolerance in type 2 diabetes. *Am J Clin Nutr* 2002; 76:1000-1006.

Milbury P, Chen C-Y, Kwak H-K, and Blumberg J. Almond skin polyphenolics act synergistically with alpha-tocopherol to increase the resistance of low-density lipoproteins to oxidation. *Free Radical Research* 2002; 36 Supp 1:78-80.

Davis P, Iwahashi CK, and Yokahama W. Whole almonds activate gastrointestinal tract anti-proliferative signaling in APCmin (Multiple Intestinal Neoplasia) mice. *FASEB Journal* 2003; 17(5):A1153.

Ren Y, Waldron KW, Pacy JF, and Ellis PR. Chemical and histochemical characterization of cell wall polysaccharides in almond seeds in relation to lipid bioavailability. Biologically active phytochemicals in food. (ed.) Pfannhauser W, Fenwick GR, and Khokhar S. Cambridge, UK. Royal Soc of Chem, 2001; 448-452.

Turnball WH, Walton J, and Leeds AR. Acute effects of mycoprotein on subsequent energy intake and appetite variables. *Am J Clin Nutr* 1993; 58(4):507-512.

Mattes R, Hollis J, Hayes D, Stunkard A. Appetite: Measurement and manipulation misgivings. *J Am Diet Assoc* 2005; 105:S87-S97.

Prior RL, et al. *J Agric Food Chem* 1998; 46:2686-2693.

Bickford PC, et al. *Society for Neuroscience Abs* 1998; 24:2157.

Agarwal S, Rao AV. Tomato lycopene and its role in human health and chronic diseases. *CMAJ* 2000; 163:739-744.

Agarwal S, Rao AV. Tomato lycopene and low density lipiprotein oxidation: a human dietary intervention study. *Lipids*. 1998; 33:981-984.

Arab L, Steck S. Lycopene and cardiovascular disease. *Am J Clin Nutr* 2000; 71(suppl); 1691S-1695S.

Bohm Y, Bitsch R. Intestinal absorption of lycopene from different matrices and interactions to other carotenoids, the lipid status, and the antioxidant capacity of human plasma. *Eur J Nutr* 1999; 38:118-125.

Ellison. Balancing the risks and benefits of moderate drinking. *Ann NY Acad Sci* 2002; 957:1.

Papamichael, et al. Red wine's antioxidants counteract acute endothelial dysfunction caused by cigarette smoking in healthy nonsmokers. *Am Heart J* 2004; 147,E5.

Volpato, et al. Relationship of alcohol intake with inflammatory markers and plasminogen activator inhibitor in well-functioning older adults. *Circulation* 2004; 109:607.

Mukamal, et al. Prospective study of alcohol consumption and risk of dementia in older adults. *JAMA* 2003; 289:1405.

Djousse, et al. Alcohol consumption and risk of intermittent claudication in the Framingham Heart Study. *Circulation*. 2000; 102:3092.

Howard, et al. Effect of alcohol consumption on diabetes mellitus: Asystematic review. *Ann Intern Med* 2004; 140:211.

Mukamal, et al. Roles of drinking pattern and type of alcohol consumed in coronary heart disease in men. *NEJM* 2003; 348;109.

Reynolds, et al. Alcohol consumption and risk of stroke: A meta analysis. *JAMA* 2003; 289:579.

Tolstrup, et al. Drinking pattern and mortality in middleaged men and women. *Addiction* 2004; 99:323.

Gordon M, Martin F, Almeida M. Antioxidant activity of hydroxytyrosol acetate compared with that of other olive oil polyphenols. *J Agric Food Chem* 2001; 49:2480-2485.

Baldioli M, Servili M, Perretti G, Montedoro G. Antioxidant activity of tocopherols and phenolic compounds of virgin olive oil. *J Am Chem Soc* 1996; 73:1589-1593.

Tsmidou M. Polyphenols and quality of virgin olive oil in retrospect. *Ital J Food Sci* 1998; 10:99-116.

Visioli F, Galli C. The effect of minor constituents of olive oil on cardiovascular disease: New findings. *Nutrition Reviews* 1998; 56(5):142-147.

Adom KK, Liu RH. Anitoxidant activity of grains. *J Agric Food Chem* 2002, 50:6182-6187.

Tucker KL. Dietary intake and coronary heart disease: A variety of nutrients and phytochemcials are important. *Current*

Treatment Options Cardiovascular Medicine 2004; 4:291-302.

Rimm, et al. Vegetable, fruit, and cereal fiber intake and risk of coronary heart disease among men. *JAMA* 1996; 274:447-451.

Mckeown, et al. Whole grain intake is favorable associated with metabolic risk factors for type 2 diabetes and cardiovascular disease. *Am J Clin Nutr* 2002; 76:390-98.

Venn BJ and Mann JL. Cereal grains, legumes, and diabetes. *Eur J Clin Nutr* 2004; May 19.

Liu S. et al. Dietary fiber intake and obesity. *National Research Newsletter* 2003; 22:12.

A Food and Taste Tour of the Sonoma Diet
California Avocado Healthy Times. California Avocado Commission, 2005.

California Avocado Information Bureau Release. New research shows avocados act as nutrient booster, August 2, 2004.

Code of Federal Regulations, Title 21: Food and Drugs. Appendix C to Part 101-Nutrition facts for raw fruits and vegetables, 2002.

Diabetes: A growing epidemic, California Avocado Healthy Times, California Avocado Commission, 2005.

Duester KC. Avocado fruit is a rich source of beta-sistosterol. *J Am Diet Assoc* 2001; 101:404-405.

Katz. Glycemic load and the risk of coronary heart disease. *Am J Clin Nutr* 2001; 73:131-132

Liu, Willet, Stampfer, et al. A prospective study of dietary glycemic load, carbohydrate intake, and risk of coronary heart disease in U.S. women. *Am J Clin Nutr* 2000; 71: 6; 1455-1461.

Salmeron J, Manson J, Stampfer J, et al. Dietary fiber, glycemic load, and risk of non insulin-dependent diabetes mellitus in women. *JAMA* 1997; 277:472-77.

Slavin J, Jacobs D, Marquart L. Whole grain consumption and chronic disease: Protective mechanisms. *Nutr Cancer* 1997; 27:14-21.

Eichholzer M, Luthy J, Gutzwiller F, Stahelin H. The role of folate, antioxidant vitamins and other constituents in fruit and vegetables in the prevention of cardiovascular disease: The epidemiological evidence. *Int J Vitam Nutr Res* 2001; 71(1):5-17.

Hemila H. Vitamin C intake and susceptibility to the common cold. *Brit J Nutr* 1997; 77, 59-72.

Whitney EN, Cataldo, CB, Rolfes, SR. Understanding normal and clinical Nutrition. Fifth Edition, Brooks Cole, 1998.

Ronzio RA. Nutritional support for the immune system. *Amer J Nat Med*, Vol. 5, No. 3.

Kris-Etherton PM, Harris WS, Appel LJ. AHA Scientific Statement: Fish consumption, fish oil, omega-3 fatty acids and cardiovascular disease. *Circulation* 2002; 106:2747.

McManus K, Antinoro L, Sacks F. A randomized controlled trial of a moderate-fat, low-energy diet compared with a low-fat, low-energy diet for weight loss in overweight individuals. *International J Obesity* 2001; 25:1-9.

Kivipelto M, et al. Body mass index, clustering of vascular risk factors, risk of dementia: A longitudinal population based study. *Neurol Bio of Aging*. Elsevior 25 (Supp 2): 2004.

Kang J, et al. Fruit and vegetable consumption and cognitive decline in women. *Neurol Bio of Aging*. Elsevior 25 (Supp 2): 2004.

American Diabetes Association. Evidence-based nutrition principles and recommendations for the treatment and prevention of diabetes and related complications. *Diabetes Care* 2002; 25 (Supp 1):S50-S60.

Hu FB, Cho E, Rexrode KM, Albert CM, Manson JE. Fish and long-chain omega-3 fatty acid intake and risk of coronary heart disease and total mortality in diabetic women. *Circulation*. 2003; 107:1852-1857.

Terpstra, A. Effect of conjugated linoleic acid on body composition and plasma lipid in humans: An overview of the literature. *Am J Clin Nutr* 2004; 79:352-61.

Belury MA. Dietary conjugated linoleic acid in health. Physiological effects and mechanisms of action. *Annu Rev Nutr* 2002; 22:505-531.

Clifton PM, et al. Trans fatty acids in adipose tissue and the food supply are associated with myocardial infarction. *J Nutr* 2004; 134:874-79.

Han SN, Leka LS, et al. Effect of hydrogenated and saturated, relative to polyunsaturated fat on immune and inflammatory responses of adults with moderate hypercholesterolemia. *J Lipid Res* 2002; 43(3):445-52.

Albers R, Bol M, Bleumink R, et al. Effects of dietary lipids on immune function in a murine sensitization model. *Br J Nutr* 2002; 88(3):291-9.

James M, et al. Dietary polyunsaturated fatty acids and inflammation mediator production. *Am J Clin Nutr* 2000; 71:343-348.

Klatsky A. Alcohol and health: How much is good for you? *Scientific American*, Feb. 2003.

Klatsky A. and Friedman G., Annotations: Alcohol and longevity. *Amer J Public Health I* 1995; 85910:16-18.

Gronbaek M, et al. Type of alcohol consumed and mortality from all causes, coronary heart disease, and cancer; *Annals of Internal Med* 2000; 133(6).

Santiago LA, Hiramatsu M, and Mori A. Japanese soybean paste miso scavenges free radicals and inhibits lipid peroxidation. *J Nutr Science* 1992; 38:297.

Hegstead DM, Ausman LM, Johnson JA, Dallal GE. Dietary fat and serum lipids: An evaluation of the experimental data. *Am J Clin Nutr* 1993; 57:875-83.

Begley, Sharon. Beyond Vitamins. *Newsweek*, April 25, 1994.

Potter SM. Overview of the proposed mechanisms for the hypocholesterolemic effect of soy. *J Nutr* 1995; 125:606S.

Alper C and Mattes R. Peanut consumption improves indices of cardiovascular disease risk in healthy adults. *J Amer Coll of Nutr* 2003; 22(2):133-141.

Dawber TR, Nickerson, et al. Eggs, serum cholesterol, and coronary heart disease. *Am J Clin Nutr* 1982; 36:617-625.

Hu FB, Stampfer MJ, Rimm EB, et al. A prospective study of egg consumption and risk of cardiovascular disease in men and women. *JAMA*; 281:1387-1394.

Wave 1

Davidson TL. Artificial sweeteners may damage diet efforts. *Int J Obesity* July 2004; 28:933-935.

Jarrett, et al. Anxiety and depression are related to autonomic nervous system function in women with irritable bowl syndrome. *Digest Dis Sci* 2003; 48(2):386-394.

Wave 2

Slavin JL, Martini PC, Jacobs D, Marquart L. Plausible mechanisms for protectiveness of whole grains. *Am J Clin Nutr* 1999; 70:459S-463S.

Liu SM, Stampfer MJ, Hu FB, Giovannucci E, Rimm E, Manson JE, Hennekens CH, Willett WC. Whole-grain consumption and risk of coronary heart disease: results from the Nurse's Health Study. *Am J Clin Nutr* 1999; 70:412-429.

Jacobs DR, Marquart L, Slavin JL, Kushi LH. Whole-grain intake and cancer: An expanded review and meta-analysis. *Nutr Cancer* 1998; 30:85-96.

Chatenoud L, Tavani A, La Vecchia C, Jacobs DR, Negri E, Levi F, Franceschi S. Whole-grain food intake and cancer risk. *Int J Cancer* 1998; 77:24-28.

Salmeron J, Aserio A, Rimm EB, Colditz, GA, Spiegelman D, Jenkins DJ, Stampfer MJ, Wing AL, Willett WC. Dietary fiber, glycemic load, and risk of NIDDM in men. *Diabetes Care* 1997; 20:545-550.

Salmeron J, Manson JE, Stampfer MJ, Colditz GA, Wing AL, Willett WC. Dietary fiber, glycemic load, and risk of non-insulin-dependent diabetes mellitus in women. *JAMA* 1997; 277,472-477.

Wu X, et al. *J Agricultural and Food Chemistry* June 2004; 52 (12): 4026-4037.

Shea T, et al. *J Nutr, Health and Aging*, 2004 March; 8:92-97.

Amer J Epidemiology 1997; 146:223-230

Klatsky A. Alcohol and health: How much is good for you? *Scientific Amer* 2003 Feb.

Klatsky A and Friedman G. Annotations: Alcohol and longevity. *Amer J Public Health I* 1995; 85910:16-18.

Clement MV, Hipara JL, Chawdhury SH, Pervaiz S. Chemopreventive agent resveratrol, a natural product derived from grapes, triggers CD95 signaling-dependent apoptosis in human tumor cells. *Blood* 1998 Aug. 1; 92(3):996-1002.

Cos P, De Bruyne T, Apers S, Vanden Berghe D, PietersL, Vlietinck AJ. Phytoestrogens: Recent developments. *Planta Medica* 2003; 69, 589-599.

Goldberg IJ, Mosca L, Piano MR, Fisher, EA. Wine and your heart [electronic version]. *Circulation* 2001 Jan. 23; 103(3): 472-475.

Additional Resources
MEDICAL JOURNAL ARTICLES
Hu FB. Walter C. Willett
Optimal diets for prevention of coronary heart disease. *JAMA* 2002 Nov; 288: 2569-2578.

Hu FB, Bronner L, Stampfer MJ, Rexrode KM, Albert CM, Hunter D; Manson JE. Fish and omega-3 fatty acid intake and risk of coronary heart disease in women. *JAMA* 2002 Apr; 287: 1815-1821.

Willett WC, et al. Diet and cancer: An evolving picture. *JAMA* 2005; 293:233-234.

Esposito, et al. Effect of a Mediterranean-style diet on endothelial dysfunction and markers of vascular inflammation in the metabolic syndrome: A randomized trial. *JAMA* 2004; 292:1440-1446.

Willett WC, et al. Reduced-Carbohydrate Diets: No role in weight management? *Ann Intern Med* 2004; 140:836-837.

Schulze and Hu. Dietary Approaches to Prevent the Metabolic Syndrome: Quality versus quantity of carbohydrates. *Diabetes Care* 2004; 27:613-614.

Din, et al. Omega-3 fatty acids and cardiovascular disease—fishing for a natural treatment. *BMJ* 2004; 328:30-35.

Jean Ferrières. The French paradox: lessons for other countries. *Heart* 2004; 90:107-111.

Hu FB. Plant-based foods and prevention of cardiovascular disease: an overview *Am. J Clin Nutr* 2003; 78:544S-551.

Fung and Hu. Plant-based diets: What should be on the plate? *Am J Clin Nutr* 2003; 78:357-358.

Hu FB. The Mediterranean Diet and Mortality—Olive Oil and Beyond. *N Engl J Med* 2003; 348:2595-2596.

Siew. Optimal diets to prevent heart disease. *JAMA* 2003; 289:1510-1510.

Bryan and McDougall. Optimal diets to prevent heart disease. *JAMA* 2003; 289:1509-1509.

Renaud S and de Lorgeril M. Wine, alcohol, platelets, and the French paradox for coronary heart disease. *Lancet* 1992; 339:1523–6.

Trichopoulos, et al. *British Medical Journal*, 2004 Apr. 8.

Joseph, et al. Reversals of age-related declines in neuronal signal transduction . . . with blueberry, spinach or strawberry dietary supplementation. *J Neuroscience* 1999 Sept. 15; 190(18): 8114-8121.

Online Articles & Websites
American Heart Association. Does a Mediterranean-style diet follow American Heart Association Guidelines? www.americanheart.org/presenter.jhtml?identifier=4644.

Barry C. The Mediterranean Diet. Nutritional News 1997 Sept. www.cheshire-med.com/services/dietary/nutrinew/mediter.html.

Visioli F. Mediterranean Diets. Linus
Pauling Institute.
http://lpi.oregonstate.edu/f-
w00/mediterr.html.

Lawson S. Linus Pauling Institute
Research Report. Diet and Optimum
Health Conference 2003 May
http://lpi.oregonstate.edu/f-
w03/dohconf.html.

Biali S. Foods that score a perfect 10:
Superfoods are simple way to fight disease, improve health. Medical Post 2005
March 22; 41(12).
www.medicalpost.com/mpcontent/arti-
cle.jsp%3Fcontent%3D20050320_160613
_3944.

WHFOODS. The World's Healthiest
Foods. www.whfoods.com/foodstoc.php.

Global Gourmet. Olive Oil History.
www.globalgourmet.com/food/egg/egg0
397/oohistory.html.

USDA MYPYRAMID.
www.mypyramid.gov.

News Author: Barclay L, CME Author:
Lie D. Mediterreanean Diet May Reduce
Mortality in Elderly. *Medscape CMF.* 2005
Apr 11.

News Author: Barclay L, CME Author:
Vega C. Fish Oil Supplements May
Increase Heart Rate Variability CME.
Medscape CME 2004 Apr 11.
http://www.medscape.com/viewarti-
cle/502801.

Diet Index

RECIPE INDEX

Y